Autistic Authors, and Autistics, and Autism in Literature: A Commentary

By Thomas D. Taylor

The author gratefully acknowledges the editorial and technical
assistance, and words of encouragement provided by Elyse
Bruce in regard to the publication of this book.

This book is dedicated to Mom, Dad, Sis, Elyse Bruce, Lewis, Doug, Angella, and Lola, with a special thanks to Elyse, for providing excellent commentary, suggestions, and constructive criticism while this work was in progress.

Table of Contents

Introduction

This book does not attempt to be scholarly in any regard, but offers some general opinions about the topic of autistic authors, and autistics and autism in literature, and gives a critique and criticism of some specific literary works. It is hoped that people interested in this subject will view this work as a point of departure from which will stem further research and investigations into the topic.

Part of this book was originally published in separate parts on the Midnight In Chicago blog (www.midnightinchicago.wordpress.com) in an article series entitled "Autistics in Literature," and those parts have been republished here with significant, and sometimes severe modifications. Verbiage has been added to the previously published material as well. Both kinds of alterations were done with the goal of making this complete publication more solid and cohesive than its parts were separately.

Why write this book in the first place?

Well, it seemed an appropriate time.

What I have been noticing is that literature that is written by, for, or about autistics seems to be deviating down a dangerous path. It seems as though autism is being portrayed in literature less as a diagnosis, and more as a minority lifestyle. Sometimes it is even portrayed as a culture or cultural imperative. If that isn't enough reason to write this book, we might consider the fact that much of what is written by "autistics" is actually being written by "self diagnosed" autistics, and no matter who is doing the writing (autistic author or self-diagnosed author), plots, characterization, and other elements, are many times being drawn and presented based on observation of "autistics" with unconfirmed diagnoses in informal venues rather than upon observations of real, diagnosed autistics in realistic or controlled settings.

As we will see in the pages to come, the distinction between "diagnosed," "misdiagnosed," and "self-diagnosed" is important, and the inspiration for autistics as they are portrayed in literature is equally important.

I will also briefly discuss other areas of literature besides fiction, such as blogging, autobiographical writing, and nonfiction.

Hopefully I will be able to demonstrate to all who read this that we are at a crucial juncture in autistic literary history. While it would be unsafe to draw any firm conclusions, or even generalizations, about autistic authors, and autistics and autism in literature at present, we *can* say that by gradations, it has grown and continues to grow out of the primitivism of its infancy, but as it matures, we can see in some instances that the motives of authors may not be entirely altruistic.

Autistic Authors, and Autistics and Autism in Literature

Before we begin discussing anything in detail, I feel the need to explain what qualifies me to even comment on literature of any kind in the first place.

Well, aside from boasting a BA in English from an accredited university, among my many different professional pursuits is writing. I have "published" in many forms, and the distribution of these various forms of publishing is equally varied.

- In elementary school, I "published" a book in a writing competition.
- In high school, I "published" comments in the school newspaper.
- In college, I "published" literary abstracts, distributing copies of my abstracts to my fellow classmates.
- I have "published" some short stories in a magazine with a worldwide circulation of 25,000 subscribers (and won an award for one of them).
- I have "published" seven paperback books (two sci-fi and five horror) worldwide and more paperbacks are on the way.
- I have "published" seven electronic files worldwide, and more are on the way.
- I have "published" a political commentary in a magazine.
- I have "published" opinion pieces in many different newspapers.

- ☐ I have "published" articles within newsletters.
- ☐ I have "published" blog articles many blogs, and some of my blog articles have been republished on other blogs.
- ☐ I have "published" podcasts that I have written and co-written.
- ☐ I have "published" lyrics that I have co-written on music CDs.
- ☐ I have "published" scripts I have written in YouTube videos.
- ☐ I have "published" comments in other people's books.
- ☐ I have given author interviews in written format.
- ☐ I have given interviews on television, answering questions using information that I had written out in advance.
- ☐ I have edited material in other people's books and short stories.

All these forms of publishing and more are commonly seen as valid, and if you are reading this book, you know that I have "published" yet again, except this time I have published nonfiction instead of fiction. As you can see, I have demonstrated a grasp not only of many different kinds of publishing, but that I can publish many different kinds of literature. One assumes that in order to be successful with one's publishing ventures, one must be reasonably educated and practiced in the different forms one publishes in, and in my case, that assumption would be correct.

In the course of one's life, one can expect to engage in publishing ventures similar things to those which I have done, but maybe not in such proliferation.

Still, that amounts to half of my credentials. The other half would pertain to autism. How am I qualified to comment on autism and autistics?

- ☐ I have a significant educational background in teaching.

- ☐ I have a significant background in educational psychology.
- ☐ I have worked with special needs children, including autistics, in the school setting.
- ☐ I have worked collaboratively and cooperatively with many school administrations.
- ☐ I have advocated for individual autistics in the school system.
- ☐ I have advocated for individual autistics in the healthcare system.
- ☐ I have advocated for groups of autistics.
- ☐ I have conducted fundraisers for philanthropic organizations that serve autistics.
- ☐ I have worked for one of the world's leading consulting firms for non-profit organizations which has had autism organizations as their clients.
- ☐ I personally know and associate with executive directors of many autism organizations.
- ☐ I have communicated with many people at UNICEF regarding the Convention on the Rights of People with Disabilities.
- ☐ I have communicated with politicians in many countries about legislation concerning autism, disabilities, and the rights of disabled people.
- ☐ I have given newspaper interviews about autism.
- ☐ I have given television interviews about autism.
- ☐ I have attended autism conventions and displayed material at them.
- ☐ I own nine online forums for people on the autism spectrum and have owned them for nearly a decade.
- ☐ I have moderated and/or administrated many more online forums.
- ☐ I maintain close ties with many owners and administrators of online forums.
- ☐ I personally know one of the creators of the Aspie Quiz.
- ☐ I have spent much time communicating and listening to parents of autistics.

- I have researched and written many podcasts on autism.
- I have written many blog articles about autism.
- My authored work has been referenced by accredited professionals.
- I have been monitoring the development of autistic political movements nearly since the popular use of the internet began.
- I have friends on the autism spectrum.

There is plenty more I could add to my resume in the publishing and autism areas, but the point by now ought to be clear: I have a substantial background in writing and a substantial background in autism.

I have been online since the earliest days of Edan Dagan's Aspergia (www.aspergia.com), when it came to the net in EZ Board format. In the beginning, there were just a very few people frequenting the Aspergia board, including me. It blossomed into a board with hundreds of members, then, over a thousand before it eventually closed. Arguably, many of the boards we see online today had their origins in Aspergia. To this day, my forum members still use one of the original IRC Aspergia chat-rooms. Very few people beside myself could tell you the true story behind the board's opening and its closure, and I will assert here without proof that much of what has been written by some authors about its closure is incorrect.

With all of this said, my "qualifications" such as they are, are secondary when we factor common sense into the equation. In other words, one does not necessarily need a background like mine to be able to see what makes "good" autistic literature and what doesn't.

If, for example, you are a parent of an autistic child, your personal experience with autism as it presents in your child will give you a baseline from which you can appreciate, critique, and criticize autism in literature. If you read extensively, you are perhaps qualified to determine what does and what does not make for good literature, or at least, good writing.

Striking reader response criticism from the equation, however, we'll look at autism and autistics in literature not from the standpoint of like or dislike, but from the standpoints of credible, or incredible, real, or unreal, believable, or unbelievable.

Having given you an idea of my background, I now want to talk to you about the backgrounds of some of those who write the autistic literature we read. What follows is not all encompassing, and should be regarded as food for thought.

But first, I need to ask two brutally honest questions.

1. How serious are you about learning more about autism as it actually presents itself?
2. How serious are you about helping a loved one who actually has autism?

My reason for asking is because – though most people won't admit to it – the answer to both of the above questions many times is "Not very." This answer holds especially true for autistics and parents of autistics. This attitude, in my opinion, is in part what allows poor authors to penetrate the literary marketplace and rise to prominence within it. As I will soon demonstrate, there really are very few authors that can be trusted to write accurately or responsibly about autism.

I hear these statements from autistics and parents of autistics everywhere we go, and particularly at autism conventions:

- "I read on Wikipedia that…"
- "I bought a tape by an autistic life coach who said that…"
- "I read a book by an autistic author…"
- "I'm here at this convention aren't I?"

For people who don't want to bury their heads in the library to find the really good reading material, they are willing to settle for less. Many people who write about autism know this, and they exploit their readers freely as a result. There is no way I can write the rest of this book without being brutally blunt and honest about this problem. I will talk for the next little while in terms of realities.

Reality Number One: Most people who have been diagnosed autistic would lose that diagnosis if they were examined by autism researchers and autism specialists.

One of the biggest scams going is the one presented and perpetuated by our school systems on the populace. I can say this because, having done my teacher training in various school districts, and having advocated for autistic students since my teacher training days, I have witnessed this scam being pulled on unsuspecting kids and parents time and time again.

If you have a child who has a behavioral problem, or if your child is a slow learner, or if your child has a mental disorder that's not easily identifiable, quantifiable, or diagnosable, your child may need assistance in the classroom, and rightfully so.

This assistance doesn't materialize out of thin air. It needs to be paid for, and the primary source for funding comes from one or more forms of government. It comes from states and/or counties if you live in the US, and it comes from counties and/or provinces, if you live in Canada and other countries. In many cases, federal funding may be available too.

Have you ever noticed that adults who apply for their own for disability benefits from the government –no matter where they live- are almost always turned down on the first try? Yet it seems that for kids, when funding is applied for by schools on their behalf, the dollars fly into school coffers.

Have you ever stopped to wonder why that is?

How does that happen?

Children get funded because schools fill out the application forms in a way that demonstrates a child is grossly developmentally challenged, and has special needs that are so expensive as to be unaffordable by the school district. An ADHD diagnosis used to get schools much of the funding they needed for a child. Now it's an autism diagnosis.

But the fact is, most of the kids diagnosed with autism these days don't have autism. It's the biggest secret kept in many school systems. The psychologist many districts have on staff is "on their payroll," so to speak. These people know exactly what to write on forms to get the funding for the schools they serve from county, state/provincial, and federal sources.

Sometimes, more than a "diagnosis" is needed, and so parents are coached about what to say to their child's pediatrician to get a secondary "diagnosis." Some parents are told something along the lines of "Have your pediatrician put XXXXXX on the form and give it back to us. We'll submit the paperwork for you."

Yes, I bet they will.

Then all of a sudden, the child in question gets an Educational Assistant, a laptop with assistive technology, a weekly pass to the Snozelen room, and a bunch of other nonsense. I say it's "nonsense" because, if a child actually *doesn't* have autism, but is diagnosed as being on the spectrum anyway, it means the school is actually wasting money and resources, and probably not properly educating that child. They are in fact shunting the child through the educational system using costly, time consuming "aids" that do nothing to actually educate.

Put another way, why would a school provide a visually impaired student with a touch screen computer when what they may really need is a Braille writer, voice readers on their computers, and a seeing eye dog?

These schools wind up socially promoting autistics and matriculating them on a tiered system of lowered expectations rather than providing proper supports for them. Given that many children who are "diagnosed" with autism are actually kids with behavioral problems, schools would be better off, in these questionable days of political correctness, forcing these misdiagnosed children to buckle down and study harder.

Parents of behaviorally challenged or special needs children are similarly victimized. Because no parent wants to admit that they are poor disciplinarians, or that they don't know how to handle a kid with special needs, schools seize on that fact, prey upon it, and use kids to gain funding which they can use to their advantage.

Why would schools do this?

For the simple reason that the school population in total has special needs kids, and providing for the *general* needs of all of them means that they can serve a wider segment of the student population than just a select few. You will find that a common complaint many parents have about educational assistants, for example, is that there are not enough of them to go around. Funding may have been obtained for a single student to sit with an EA for the entire school day, yet, for some inexplicable reason, this EA is made to divide his or her time between two or more students. Yet as hard as a full time EA is to come by, a school may have a Snozelen room. This indoor playground is expensive to build, and requires huge allocations of space in an age when many of our schools are overcrowded and underfunded.

How many times do we see a school push its students to sell candy bars to raise money for itself while students' needs go unaddressed even as a Snozelen room sits empty?

For schools and districts that are guilty of this financial shell game, it's all just a show. "We're doing something for our autistic students," is the message these schools are trying to get across.

But most of the kids they are saying are autistic really aren't autistic at all.

Reality Number Two: Many children and adults who see these misdiagnosed "autistics" self-diagnose themselves, and many misdiagnosed and self-diagnosed autistics use their supposed diagnoses to take you for all you're worth.

While we can understand how someone can be misdiagnosed, can we really believe that an autism diagnosis can be *faked*? After all, for self-diagnosed "autistics" to "look the part" on demand they have to appear autistic to anyone who may question their diagnosis.

Can it be done?

Yes.

As proof, I offer Dustin Hoffman and Claire Danes, who played Rainman in <u>Rainman</u>, and Temple Grandin in <u>Temple Grandin</u> respectively on the big screen. While any moviegoer knows that people who portray other people on the screen are just actors, both Hoffman and Danes convinced millions of people around the world that they were watching an accurate portrayal of autism. Furthermore, in the case of <u>Rainman</u>, Kim Peek, the autistic man upon whom Rainman was based, shares only a few qualities with Hoffman's character. Thus while Hoffman's Rainman isn't exactly a lie or a fraud, it's not exactly true either.

Hoffman and Danes didn't instantly fall into their roles. Rather, they were coached, and told how to behave. In fact, Hoffman was actually coached by Temple Grandin. It is not so much of a stretch, then, to posit that, like Hoffman and Danes, anyone could learn how to imitate someone with autism and carry out this act for a lifetime.

Realistically speaking, however, living a lie for one's whole life is not easy, and is not something someone would likely do. Yet, when you factor in that many self-diagnosed people naturally have some traits similar to those displayed by real autistics, faking might not be so hard.

If we can accept that self-diagnosed autistics can fake their diagnosis, how then, do they, along with misdiagnosed autistics, take advantage of unsuspecting consumers?

They do it by making tapes, giving lectures, and writing books.

Let me explain to you using a metaphor why mis-diagnosis and self-diagnosis can be detrimental to oneself and others outside the psychological and medical realm.

Pretend that you've just bought a house and your kitchen is in poor shape.

You want it replaced and you solicit bids from contractors.

The first one arrives, you tell him what you want done, he takes some measurements, and returns to you with a bid of $25,000.00, explaining to you that the job will take four men six weeks to do. The huge cost is primarily attributable to the price of the quality materials he will be using, and the fact that the plumbing and electrical are going to need to be updated. He gives you a list of references, which you set aside pending further bids.

The next contractor comes along, a woman this time, and says she can do it for $23,000.00. Being a woman-owned business, she has the added benefit of getting certain grants which keep her operational costs low. She tells you that the plumbing is indeed substandard, but that rather than sub-contract the electrical, she has an in-house electrician who can save you money on that part of the job.

Encouraged by the fact that the cost of the project seems to be going down, you ask for bids from other companies, but to your disappointment, they all come in between $22,500.00 and - my gosh- $27,000.00, and worse, it will take anywhere from five weeks to *nine* weeks to get the job done, depending on which contractor you go with, and depending on when the cabinets - which have to be made to order- come in.

But then, along comes your savior, a contractor who says he can do the whole job for $10,000.00 in three weeks or less. His reasons for the low cost seem sensible to you. The cabinets you are ordering are actually ones that are soon to be discontinued by the manufacturer. Not only can he get them to you at wholesale prices, but because he knows the owner of the company, he can get them for you for even less than wholesale. And they don't need to be "made to order" either because they are already "in stock" and waiting to be liquidated. In fact, the manufacturer will be giving you a low price because he wants to make space for new inventory.

Regarding the plumbing and electrical, yes, they need to be updated, but this contractor tells you the parts are standard, and he has the necessary parts left over from other jobs that he can use. So in reality, the parts are already paid for and you're getting them for nothing.

As for how long it's going to take to get done, it will take three weeks because there will be no wait for the cabinets to arrive, plain and simple. Figure one day for demolition, one day for re-framing, one day to install the electrical, one day for the plumbing rough in, one day for inspection on both of them, one day to put up the sheet rock and plaster, one day for the floors, one day to install the cabinets, one day to install the counters, one day to install the appliances, one day for cleanup, and there you go. That's eleven days of actual work with four days to allow for anything unexpected.

Best of all, one of the guys on his crew is an "artisan in training." Apprentices of this type are paid less, he explains, and the contractor is willing to pass on this reduced labor cost to you. He gives you a short list of references.

Hardly believing your luck, you call the references and discover that his customers are completely satisfied, never realizing that the people you are calling are friends and relatives of his.

You go with this person and by the end of five weeks (the job took longer than expected) you have a new kitchen!

The problem is, things aren't quite right. The cabinets look like the ones you wanted, but they are actually made of medium density fiberboard with wood veneer. They are not hung properly. Some of the doors swing open on their own. The hardware isn't always symmetrical either. The plumbing is a bit leaky, and one of the outlets wobbles in its box. Plus, sometimes when you are cooking something in the oven and have the dishwasher running, a circuit cuts out.

Speaking of the dishwasher, it keeps having problems. It seems to you that you've spent more money getting the dishwasher fixed than the thing cost in the first place. The contractor had told you the appliances he got you were top quality, but he must have picked a lemon out of the tree when he got you that dishwasher.

The floor squeaks, and some of the gaps between the slats are a bit too wide. You can see where the plasterer forgot to sand some of the seams on the walls, and, well...there are a lot of things wrong with the job.

For years, however, you try and convince yourself and others that your decision to go with the bad contractor was the right one, that you got the better end of the deal, and that your kitchen was exactly what you wanted.

But finally, when a pipe bursts, and some other problems become more than you can handle with your limited do it yourself knowledge, you decide to call in a bonafide contractor to do the job right. Adjusting for the rate of inflation, the job will now cost a whopping $42,000.00, which is much more than the $25,000.00 you had hoped for.

There are many reasons for this price jump.

Because the previous contractor sawed through some floor joists to do the plumbing rough in, part of your kitchen floor has no support at all. Worse, the leaky pipes rotted out part of the underlayment, which caused mold damage. So now you have to get a special person in to get rid of the mold, and, if you want the floor to be repaired seamlessly, you'll have to rip out the floor down to the joists. That might be a good thing anyway, because if the contractor can see how the wiring was done, he might get to the bottom of the problem with the circuit cutting out so often.

The cabinet doors opened on their own sometimes because they were nailed into the soffits, not screwed. Over time, gravity caused them to hang crooked. This problem could be easily corrected with screws except that the soffits need to be removed anyway because they were built with poor engineering specs and are really incapable of supporting fully loaded cabinets.

By the way, your appliances weren't new, they were actually "refurbished" which might explain why you had to get your dishwasher fixed so many times.

And...and...

You get the picture, but there are still some things you don't understand. Why was the plumbing leaking all of this time? Why didn't the inspector find the leak, and why didn't the inspector notice the plumber had cut the floor joists for the rough in?

As your contractor gets to work, he answers your questions for you.

Your contractor tells you that he took it upon himself to check city records and discovered that not only are there no records of the plumbing and electrical inspections, but that there were never any permits filed for the original job either. The permits that were posted in the front window were probably fake, and the "inspectors" were probably just people the contractor had on his payroll. That might explain why one of the electrical circuits cut out now and then. The stove should have been on its own circuit instead of hooked up to the one that ran the fridge, the dishwasher, and all the outlets.

The point is, some times when we think we know better than professionals, we really don't, and what we think we know can actually hurt us in the long run.

A person can self-diagnose themselves with autism in a number of different ways.

1. They may have a friend on the spectrum, and identify with some of his or her symptoms, and diagnose themselves.
2. They may read a newspaper or magazine and see themselves as being similar to the people mentioned in the newspaper or magazine, and diagnose themselves.
3. They may identify with a fictitious autistic character in a book, magazine, television show, movie, etc, and they diagnose themselves.
4. They may read the DSM IV (Diagnostic and Statistical Manual of Mental Disorders, 4th edition), DSM V (Diagnostic and Statistical Manual of Mental Disorders, 5th edition), or ICD 10 (International Statistical Classification of Diseases and Related Health Problems, 10th edition) and identify with the "symptoms" listed therein, and diagnose themselves.
5. They may read a study and see themselves as being similar to the test subjects, and diagnose themselves.
6. They may take a comment from a diagnosed person or doctor as being a diagnosis (e.g. "You share a trait or two with people on the autism spectrum.").
7. They may transfer a diagnosis from a family member, or relative to themselves. (e.g., "My brother has a diagnosis, and I share many of his 'Aspie Traits' so I must have Asperger Syndrome too, only much milder.").
8. They may take an informal online test or quiz, (e.g. The Aspie Quiz) which may suggest that they might have Asperger Syndrome, and diagnose themselves. However, they may ignore any caution that says only a professional clinician can make an informed diagnosis.
9. They may take a respected online assessment test or quiz and diagnosis themselves (e.g. The Australian Scale for Asperger Syndrome by M.S. Garnett and Tony Attwood) and diagnose themselves. However,

they ignore any caution that says only a professional clinician can make an informed diagnosis. **Note:** Oftentimes people who use this online diagnostic test will stretch the truth and say things like "A professionally developed and recognized test diagnosed me with Asperger Syndrome," or "Tony Attwood diagnosed me," or "I was professionally diagnosed."

10. They may be made an "honorary autistic" by other people who are or who believe themselves to be on the spectrum, and consider this to be an informal diagnosis.

There are many more ways people can self-diagnose, but my point ought to be clear: Self-diagnosis is specious and unreliable. Aside from that, a self-diagnosis is not recognized as an official diagnosis by medical professionals.

People will self-diagnose themselves with autism, but if they are told repeatedly by professional medical personnel that they don't have it, and what they do have is something else, they would be wise to listen to the diagnosticians rather than themselves, and if, after being told by many doctors that they are not autistic, and they find one that tells them they *are* autistic, they would be wise to suspect whether or not what that one doctor is telling them is true.

As I have said, I have been circulating in the autism community online since just about the time the internet became widely used.

Sixteen years ago I was seeing kids joining autism forums who were saying things like "I've been diagnosed with Oppositional Defiant Disorder, but I think I'm really autistic because people don't understand me. I'm going in for testing to get checked for autism." Invariably, people like these reported that autism was ruled out, but, interestingly enough, more diagnoses were tacked on that were behaviorally related.

One woman specifically, who now claims to be an "autism warrior" was diagnosed as being psychopathic, and this diagnosis, to my knowledge, remains unchanged to the present day. "Autism" as far as I know, was never her diagnosis, yet she claims to be autistic.

These "posers," many of whom have been repeatedly -and in no uncertain terms- told by board certified medical professionals that they are not by any stretch of the imagination autistic (regardless of whether or not they were previously "diagnosed" by school psychologists) are now giving lectures, making tapes and videos, writing books, and billing themselves as "autistic life coaches."

There is an avid critic of the Midnight In Chicago blog who claims to be autistic. He has *not* to my knowledge been diagnosed autistic, but *has* stated elsewhere that he has been diagnosed with bipolar disorder. This person has a video-blog and a series of other blogs designed to tell anyone who will listen about how autism has impacted his (or her – I'm not going to spill the beans on who this person is) life, and what people can do to make life easier for autistics. This person has written one "book" (never published, except for free distribution in the form of an electronic file) and has been trying to write other books for many years now.

Supposedly, according to this person, he has one "novel" that is being "considered by agents" whatever that means. Whether or not the "novel" and the "book" are one and the same, I do not know. But I must say that I find the assertion about agents misleading. Having once been in the market for agents, I've spoken with a few of them about their services and what they could potentially do for me. I know that before they would solicit my writing, they would "consider" whether or not what I had to submit was worth soliciting. To say that an agent is "considering" something is like saying Readers Digest is "considering" a joke for publication. Sure your piece of writing is being "considered." Yours and many others.

But when it comes to publishing something as significant as a "novel," I don't think it is acceptable to imply that it is on the road to being published when it hasn't even passed initial muster.

There is another "autistic" person who was living in (his or her) parents' basement until recently, who lectures, makes videos, and writes books. The books he publishes tell autistics about how to make successes out of their lives. Autistics and parents of autistics alike buy into his spiel, probably never realizing how unsuccessful the person is they are buying the books from.

People who admit to never being diagnosed are not exempt from being deceptive when writing about autism. There is a person who bills himself or herself as a "doctor," and who has incorporated and referenced unproven junk science in one of his or her publications (which was a work of nonfiction). I have not yet seen this person produce either a medical license or a doctorate degree to prove his or her credentials. Certainly, this person, doctor or no, doesn't appear to be able differentiate between peer-reviewed studies, and quackery. Readers, however, can expect to pay an impressive premium for the book.

A brief note about self-publishing...

There are times when it may be advantageous for an author to self-publish. If an author is well-versed in writing, formatting text, editing, proofreading, illustrating, photographing, designing a cover jacket, and promoting, and if the author has a knowledge of copyright law, he or she may be able to create a book from cover to cover, doing everything from the copyright notice to the afterword. Skilled authors can expect to reap higher profits on books they assemble on their own.

However, if an author is less skilled, he or she may hire an editor and/or proofreader, and/or an illustrator, and/or a photographer, and/or a graphic artist, and/or a lawyer to help them through the process of bringing their book to publication. These costs must be recouped, and the costs are ultimately built into the price of the book. Other things which may inflate the cost of the book are things like promotion, and hiring someone to manage the tax ramifications of sales and profit.

There are vanity presses, where a person can pay to have a number of books (paperback or hardback) printed. The person can then sell them for whatever price they choose. Similar to vanity presses are online self-publishing venues like Amazon and Createspace.com. There too, you can upload a file of your book and this book will be published in electronic and paperback format on Amazon.com, and in paperback format on Createspace.com. As with regular vanity presses, the author sets the price on his or her products.

In all three cases, there may be costs involved that are incurred from the earliest stages of production all the way up to press time. This is due to certain requirements imposed on the author by the publisher. There may be certain requirements for formatting, for example, and if the author is not particularly savvy with meeting those requirements, he may have to pay the publisher to do the formatting for him. Both Amazon.com and Createspace.com offer services to assist an author with certain stages of publication, and they charge a price in return for these services.

Both Amazon.com and Creatspace.com offer limited free distribution channels to the author, as well as additional distribution channels for a fee, and they offer the author anywhere between a 30% royalty and 70% royalty on all sales, depending on where and how the product is distributed.

All things considered, if an author has done all that is necessary to bring a book to publication on either Amazon.com or Createspace.com they should be able to charge as much for a book as the major publishing houses do, and still make a good profit. If you see, for example, a 370 page book drafted in 10 point font, measuring 5" x 8" costing $12.99 to $16.99, for paperback, and anywhere from .99 cents to $4.99 in kindle format, that may be a fair price. But if you see an author charging double or triple that price, it may be price gouging.

Content is of course the most important part of any book. I have seen books on autism that look very classy on the outside, but inside, there may be little more than a compilation of material randomly acquired from the net, virtually copied and pasted, with only slight modifications or added commentary. These books may sell for much more than they are worth.

Let the buyer beware.

Minor and major publishing houses can be guilty of price gouging too.

Minor and major publishing houses will usually do a professional job in bringing a book to market. Most work will be done in-house. Seldom will any work be subcontracted. This keeps production costs low. However, autism is a subject matter that can best be described as satisfying a small market. Thus for a publisher to recoup the cost of the initial expenditure of bringing the book to market, they will charge more for a book about autism than they would charge for a book with a topic that is more likely to draw a broader range of consumers, such as a book about aging and Alzheimer's.

The advantage to having a minor or major publishing house publish a book is that an author will usually get paid according to some kind of contract and/or royalty, so income is almost assured. Additionally, an author's work may be better promoted and/or more widely distributed than if the author went the self-publishing route.

However, as will be mentioned again later, a publisher's job is not necessarily to evaluate the content of a book on the basis of whether or not it is factual or valid. In a time when print is dying, publishers these days may look at a book from three different vantage points:

1. Is the book going to be something that people will want to read?
2. Is the book something that will sell?
3. Is the book something that's not going make the publisher legally liable to someone in some way?

Thus as a consumer, you could buy a book about autism from a reputable publisher at a very high price and the content may be worthless. Further, given that authors know that books about autism are specialty books, authors may demand that a book's price be set higher than the price set for other books. In this way, they can add to their own income, while hiding this greedy "fee" within the price of the book.

A message from myself to my readers:

This book will be offered at a reasonable price so that it might reach the widest possible audience.

Reality Number Three: Many self-diagnosed autistics aren't interested in helping you.

These are sometimes the ones who write books about their supposed "autistic experience." Their target audience is gullible people who are likely to think after the last page is turned: "It's so amazing that they overcame their autism!"

Well, anyone can overcome autism if they've never had autism in the first place.

I'll make a couple of points here so that my message to you is perfectly clear:

1. If someone is trying to sell you something, why would you buy it from them if their credentials are in question? If they are willing to lie to you about their credentials, what else are they willing to lie to you about?

2. If you are autistic, or the caregiver of an autistic person, you are not being helped by books written by misdiagnosed or self-diagnosed autistics who may not have autism at all. So don't read them.

3. If you think that buying a book, or attending a lecture, or watching a video is going to give you everything you need to help you or someone else with autism, then you're kidding yourself. Medical researchers have spent decades studying autism, and while much progress has been made, there is still much to be learned. If you want to truly learn more about autism, then learn what researchers have learned. Study hard, in other words.

4. Whether they are writing fiction or nonfiction, misdiagnosed or self-diagnosed autistics might not be basing their works in facts and research, but in conjecture and supposition.

To build a little on that last point, www.aspergia.com has of course has been closed many years now, but its staying power in the memories of those who frequented the board remain a testament to Edan Dagan's ability as a board owner and administrator, and also his ability as a writer of fiction. The Aspergian Mythos (which will be discussed a little more later on) was so powerfully written that many have come to accept this entertaining read as theory and hypothesis when in fact it was only meant to be fantasy and fun.

Were he a different kind of person, Dagan might have tried to pass off fiction as fact.

Reality Number Four: Many diagnosed autistics aren't interested in helping you either.

These types of people, who may indeed have professional diagnoses, publish books (both fiction and nonfiction) and go on the lecture circuit. There they may tell you about their experiences, and they will tell you how they overcame challenges, but what many of their words boil down to is "Look at me! Look at what I did! And read my books on account of me being so extraordinary!"

There is no reason why you should care about what a diagnosed person has done or accomplished any more than you should care about what someone without a diagnosis has done or accomplished.

That autism *can be* an obstacle for some people is a fact, but it is not an obstacle for *everyone* who has been diagnosed with it. Do not be swayed or influenced merely by the fact that someone with autism has done something, instead be swayed and influenced only if what they have done is truly remarkable.

Aside from that, one thing researchers will tell you is that if you've seen one autistic, you've seen one autistic. And so, what one autistic may tell you will be different from what someone else will tell you. Reading about one person's experience will be interesting, but it will be different from another person's experience. If you are reading a fictional publication published by an autistic, remember that the author of that publication will be telling you a story as they have composed it. Their worldview will surely be incorporated into that story, but it will be a different worldview than another autistic's.

If they are writing self help or how to books, remember that what may be helpful for one autistic may have the opposite effect on another. Only sound medical research which has been peer-reviewed can be relied upon to provide beneficial information to autistics and caregivers of autistics.

One must also consider that what you hear from a lecturer or writer will be honed and embellished, or else it wouldn't be interesting to the paying audience or customer. In either case, you are paying someone to tell you what you want to hear. The world is full of rags to riches stories, for example, but how many people publish their stories, and how many have you read? When you have read such stories, what was it that caused you to pick up the book in the first place? What was the selling point that got you to take money out of your pocket and put it into someone else's? Would you read an autobiographical account of an autistic you've never heard of, and if so, why? What makes that person's story more relevant and insightful than any other? Just the fact that they are diagnosed with autism may not be enough.

If that same autistic publishes fiction, or nonfiction, what makes that literature worth buying? That it was written by an autistic makes it notable, but does the fiction or nonfiction stand on its own as good literature?

Reality Number Five: Whether they are diagnosed or self-diagnosed, many autistics are just as uneducated as you are, and are not reliable sources for opinions or information on autism.

They may not even be qualified to talk about their own experiences. This principle holds true whether you are reading their nonfiction or fiction.

I can speak to this point from personal experience.

I am a published author. I have seven books in print, and another (this one) will be published shortly. I have sold my books in both electronic and paperback format to many people.

This success has caused people to accept what I have to say without stopping to think about whether I am qualified to say it.

Fans often come up to me and ask for my autograph, and though I am happy to give it to them, and thankful that they have bought my books, I have to ask myself why they would want my autograph at all. I am a person, just like they are. The only difference between myself and them is that I have chosen writing as a profession. If I were a plumber, would they be asking for my autograph because I can fix their bathroom sinks? If I were an accountant, would they ask for my autograph because I could sort out their assets and liabilities for them?

One of my personal friends wanted me to autograph some of my books for her and I asked her why. She said it's because I'm a "famous" author, and she's never known a famous author before. Secretly, I laughed. I have known that friend for fifteen years now –long before I published anything except for a few short stories. She didn't ask for my autograph *then*. It's only *now* that I'm "famous" that she's asking for my autograph.

I am just an average everyday working stiff who writes stories, novellas, novels, magazine articles, and nonfiction books, and publishes them. I'm nothing special. I know telling you these things is not a good thing to do from a marketing standpoint, but I have to be honest so that your mind is not clouded with misconceptions about me. I believe that in order for you to have faith in what I am telling you, I have to show you who I am.

Fortunately for you, whenever I publish something about autism, I research the subject I am writing about extensively. What I tell you, or what I quote, is information gleaned from published studies where people have done research that has been peer-reviewed, or else I am giving you information that has been gotten from reputable books and periodicals.

And that is what *you* should do to. Don't read what I write! Go to the library and read up on autism yourself. That way you too can get the information you are seeking straight from researchers.

Quit putting your faith in *people's opinions*, and put your faith in *researched and established fact.*

But if you are going to put your faith in other people's writing, then you should expect they are going to provide you with some disclosure. Who are they? Where are they getting their information from? How do *they* know that what they are saying is true? Is what they are telling you congruent with what researchers and clinicians have discovered?

Elyse Bruce, the brainchild behind Midnight In Chicago (www.midnightinchicago.com), is an author, a singer, a songwriter, and many other things. To me, first and foremost, she is just another person like myself. But if either of us was less moral than we are, we would build ourselves up into icons to be worshiped, and we would use our celebrity status to sell you things that may not be good for you to buy.

These days in the autism world, people will say anything about themselves to get you to buy what they're selling.

If someone said, "I'm autistic. I have a twin with autism. *And* I carried an Olympic torch" should you be wowed by that send up?

I would look at those statements and say, "So what?"

Because a person is autistic, and has a twin with autism, is that enough to qualify that person to speak about autism? Someone might be diagnosed with autism, but what does that person know about its origins, its presentation, its treatment or lack thereof? And what does carrying an Olympic torch have to do with autism? Would it even matter much if the person had competed in the Olympics?

If I wanted to make myself bigger than what I am I could tell people about the "famous" people I know, and that I once shook hands with Bozo the Clown during the Grand March at the end of a Bozo's Circus episode!

I'd be telling the truth...but so what?

What does any of that have to do with autism?

Reality Number Six: Many of the "facts" about autism that you read in books written by misdiagnosed or self-diagnosed autistics are erroneous, or they are suppositions. Likewise, autism as it is depicted in fiction is oftentimes equally suspect.

For you to appreciate what I am saying, you have to admit to yourself that as much as you would like to believe that there are quick or easy solutions to problems faced by autistics, there are no quick or easy solutions. Yet lecturers and authors of books would like you to believe otherwise.

If there were quick and easy treatments –and if there were "cures" for autism- medical professionals would prescribe them, insurance would pay for them, they would be offered so broadly that they would be inexpensive, and the rate of autism diagnoses would be declining rather than expanding.

People who claim they have a secret treatment or cure for autism prey on people's hopes and ignorance. They use their audience's gullibility to their advantage. For just a little money – or a lot – the "cure" can be yours.

It's interesting to see the "cheap" and "expensive" factions go at each other. Those who believe in inexpensive "cures" follow authors and lecturers who, "out of the goodness of their hearts" and "of great expense to themselves" offer treatments and "cures" at dirt cheap prices.

But the other faction will say that nothing ever comes cheap.

The more this second group of people pay for treatments and cures, the better they feel about themselves. For many of these folks, it is too traumatic to admit that there is no cure for autism, or else they don't want to admit that they are too lazy to read real research, or that they are incapable of understanding bonafide research and proven techniques.

Many researchers will tell you that if you spend years upon years working intensively will fully autistic people, you can increase their level of functioning. But let's admit it, how many parents and caregivers really want to put in all that effort?

But if they spend lots of money on books, DVDs and quack cures, it makes them *look* like they are putting in a lot of effort. How many times have we heard from these people "I exhausted my life savings on chelation and XXXX XXXX lecture series!"?

Diagnosed, misdiagnosed, and self-diagnosed authors who tell their life stories, or who write fiction, often just want to get in on the bonanza. To this end, they may indeed include reputable facts about autism...but they may mix them in with "facts" which have been discredited. They do this to make themselves and their arguments sound more plausible.

One common theme in "autistic" fiction and nonfiction, for example, is that people who have tried to understand autistics have the most success with them. While this tends to be true from a clinical perspective, it is also true that what many misdiagnosed and self diagnosed "autistic" authors are *really* asserting -and this is going to sound harsh- is that if you let them be the way they are, they are more likely to be less of a burden on their loved ones and on society. What they are underhandedly advocating for is a license to do whatever they want, whether it is legal or illegal, moral or immoral, ethical or unethical, and they are advocating for this freedom primarily because their *real* diagnoses, which may not involve autism at all, compels them to misbehave.

As we can discern from watching people who have real autism diagnoses, if they have problems operating in society, it is usually because their symptomology acts as a hindrance to their success. They do not often act in illegal, immoral, unethical, or criminal ways as the result of personal choice, or by compulsion, the exception to the rule being when a perseverative interest becomes so pervasive as to cause an autistic to act in a manner that goes against his or her best interest.

But I have seen people online who claim to be autistic (and who have admitted privately that they are *not* on the spectrum) say that they shoplift smoke pot, drive above the speed limit, engage in partner swapping, etc., because they are autistic, and because their perseverative interests compel them to do what they do. Many of these people hold positions on the board of directors for autistic advocacy organizations. Some of them have written books.

All of them should be ignored. They are not qualified to write about autism, and unless they educated themselves about autism - and their own diagnoses (which are *not* autism) - they will never be qualified to write about autism.

You, as a consumer, should avoid any product that comes from people like these, and if you cannot tell who is who, then it may be best not to buy anything from anyone who claims to be autistic at all until you are better informed.

Another thing to consider is that when facts are presented, even by honest and earnest people, you would do well to be skeptical. If a study is quoted, it is best to read the study yourself to find out what it says exactly. Learn the difference between mean and average. Learn what an error ratio is. Learn what a control group and a placebo are. Learn what "valid" means. Learn what size sample is needed for a valid conclusion to be drawn.

I have taken a course in educational measurement, and am able to interpret to some degree whether or not a study is a good one, but even this knowledge does not negate the fact that I have no medical training whatsoever. I am therefore only partly qualified to interpret medical study results. With this said, it is doubtful that people without training, or with partial training, diagnosed, misdiagnosed, or self-diagnosed, can interpret study results with any degree of confidence. So you should not accept what is told to you at face value, especially when what they are telling you is about such an important topic like autism.

Reality Number Seven: Yes, there may be a conspiracy, and it has permeated autistic fiction and nonfiction.

There are "political": factions in the autism world. For me to list them all out would require a book in itself, but I will provide a short list of the most influential factions so you can begin to see how it is that I can make the seemingly paranoid assertion that there are conspiracies afoot.

"Autistics" may be any one of the following:

- ☐ Diagnosed
- ☐ Misdiagnosed
- ☐ Self-diagnosed
- ☐ In the process of getting a diagnosis
- ☐ Seeking a diagnosis
- ☐ Wannabee

The factions begin to emerge with this area of classification. One faction will oftentimes snub another that they consider inferior. Alliances change depending on who is sparring with whom. Two parties which often fight against one another are diagnosed and self-diagnosed autistics. Many diagnosed autistics feel that self-diagnosed autistics should get real diagnoses, rather than ride on the coattails of diagnosed autistics. Further, self-diagnosed autistics are many times people who have been examined repeatedly and have failed multiple times to meet the criteria for autism, yet they still continue to believe themselves to be autistics. However, despite their differences, diagnosed and self-diagnosed autistics will often join forces to put down wannabees. Self-diagnosed people are especially interested in subduing wannabees because many self-diagnosed people are wannabees themselves. Whereas wannabees are honest about never being diagnosed, self-diagnosed autistics may not be.

Those autistics who *are* diagnosed may be diagnosed with one of the following, according to the DSM IV (Diagnostic and Statistical Manual of Mental Disorders, 4th edition.):

- Autism
- Asperger Syndrome
- Childhood Disintegrative Disorder
- Rhett Syndrome
- Pervasive Developmental Disorder Not Otherwise Specified

There are some autistics who believe themselves to be diagnosed with more than one form of autism, but psychiatrists state clearly that a person may only be diagnosed with one form. If a person has been labeled with two different kinds of diagnosis, it is because their specific diagnosis is undetermined, and/or the current diagnosis vacates the previous. Additionally, it is not uncommon for a diagnosis to be changed throughout an autistic person's life depending on which doctor they are seeing, or how functional they may appear to the diagnosing physician during evaluative periods.

Diagnosed autistics might be:

☐ High-functioning
☐ Low-functioning

But some can be:

☐ Capable of functioning adequately in society
☐ Incapable of functioning adequately in society
☐ Educably mentally handicapped

They may also have:

☐ Co-morbid diagnoses
☐ Allergies
☐ Synesthesia

Those on the autism spectrum who are capable of making their feelings and needs known:

☐ May want to be treated
☐ May not want to be treated
☐ May want to be cured
☐ May not want to be cured

Of those who are diagnosed, misdiagnosed, self-diagnosed, in the process of getting a diagnosis, seeking a diagnosis, or are wannabees, some:

☐ Believe that autism is caused by vaccines
☐ Believe that autism is caused by mercury poisoning
☐ Believe that autism is caused by "Big Pharma" "vaccinating" or injecting people with autism (Please note that some people will use the term "vaccinate" and "inject" interchangeably in this context.)
☐ Believe that autism is caused by government "vaccinating" or injecting people with autism (Please note that some people will use the term

"vaccinate" and "inject" interchangeably in this context.)

- Believe that autism is caused by genetics
- Believe that autism is the result of recessive Neanderthal genes becoming active
- Believe that autistics manifest genes that will eventually become active for everyone when the next phase of human evolution is complete.
- Believe that autistics are alien-human hybrids
- Support ABA therapy
- Are against ABA therapy
- Support Chelation therapy
- Are against Chelation therapy
- Support gluten-free therapy
- Are against gluten-free therapy
- Support "Floortime"
- Are against "Floortime"
- Support electroshock therapy
- Are against electroshock therapy
- Support restraints
- Are against restraints
- Support Institutionalization
- Are against Institutionalization
- Support an autism registry
- Are against an autism registry
- Support sterilization of autistics
- Are against sterilization of autistics
- Support a genetic test for autism
- Are against a genetic test for autism
- Support weeding autistics out of the human genome through selective abortion
- Are against weeding autistics out of the human genome through selective abortion
- Support abortion
- Support abortion, but not selective abortion
- Are against abortion
- Believe themselves to have synesthesia
- Do not believe themselves to have synesthesia

I will take a brief break here to mention why having or not having synesthesia is important. Synesthesia is a blending of senses. A person may be able to see colors when listening to music, for example. This interesting trait or co-morbidity, call it what you will, is thought by some "autistics" to be a "super power" or alternatively, a sign that autistics and autistics alone are entering the next stage of evolution. Others see it as a supernatural, or occult like power similar to ESP, déjà vu, or the ability to predict the future.

As a parenthetical discussion: Adding to this concept of autism as an evolutionary process, in my opinion, is/was The Aspergian Mythos, a fictional, fanciful, and fantastic idea created by Edan Dagan, and posted on his Aspergia website (www.aspergia.com) back when the site was still in existence. As I understand it, The Aspergian Mythos was never meant to be a theory or hypothesis about the origins and future of autism, but meant to be an entertaining "what if." Having read the mythos, people could then join the Aspergia message board and chat room and become part of "Aspergia" and its "culture." Yet some people familiar with The Aspergian Mythos have adapted it as a theory or hypothesis nearly to the point where they believe in it.

Having been the founder of Aspergia, some would say that Dagan (who always wanted to be known as "Edan") has become a mythical figure and cultural leader. He, his site, and his mythos have been discussed in various online and offline conversations and publications, and in many of these, Edan is revered as though he is a cultural icon, his site is spoken about as though it was a physical (as opposed to virtual) place, and the mythos is discussed in philosophical and even political terms.

Most reminiscences about the board are fond and favorable, with some former members recalling feelings of genuine sadness and sorrow when Edan closed the board and chat, as though a real place was being shuttered. Many said that the Edan approved successor boards did not have quite the same "feel" as Aspergia.

People who populated the original board and used its chat oftentimes refer to themselves as "Aspergians." It is a made up name that is fast growing into popular acceptance by many who were never members of the board at all. Further, there has been some resentment by actual former members of the Aspergia board toward people who call themselves Aspergians, but who were never members of the board.

To make matters more confusing is the Aspergia "hierarchy." Are you a "true" Aspergian *only* if you were a member of the original Aspergia board? Or could you be an Aspergian if you were never a member of Edan's board, but were a member of one of Edan's approved successor boards after www.aspergia.com's closure?

Most confusing of all was the rivalry between some Aspergia successor boards, and, in one instance, a "coup" where a successor board owner claimed the board had been "stolen" by an administrator!

It all makes for an interesting study in "autistic culture" if such a thing can be said to exist, although if you have ever participated in some of the disputes, you will have found that they can get quite combative.

To return to the subject of autistic factions, of those who are diagnosed, misdiagnosed, self-diagnosed, in the process of getting a diagnosis, seeking a diagnosis, or are wannabees, some:

- Support the neurodiversity movement
- Are against the neurodiversity movement
- Like neurotypicals
- Hate neurotypicals
- Hate neurotypicals but support the neurodiversity movement

Further explanation is required here. The neurodiversity movement as I understand it believes in universal acceptance of everyone, no matter what their diagnosis might be. Neurotypicals or "NTs" are people within the bell curve of society and who are commonly considered "the norm." The autism community has usurped the meaning of the word to mean people without an autism diagnosis.

Continuing once again, of those who are diagnosed, misdiagnosed, self-diagnosed, in the process of getting a diagnosis, seeking a diagnosis, or are wannabees, some:

- ☐ Support the idea that autism is a diagnosis
- ☐ Support the idea that autism is a difference, not a diagnosis
- ☐ Support the idea that autism is a disease, and not a difference or a diagnosis
- ☐ Support the idea that autism is a mental disorder
- ☐ Support the idea that autism is none of the above, but that autistics are really a minority group
- ☐ Support the idea that autistics are a separate race

Depending on what they believe, people who are diagnosed, misdiagnosed, self-diagnosed, in the process of getting a diagnosis, seeking a diagnosis, or wannabees, may ally themselves for or against autism charities, organizations, and self-advocacy groups. They may also ally themselves with or fight against certain government organizations. The biggest charity that many love to love and love to hate seems to be Autism Speaks. Autism charities, autism organizations, and autistic self-advocacy groups may or may not incorporate any of the values listed above and many that are not listed here. These charities, groups, and organizations may or not be as firm or as fickle about their beliefs and values as its membership. Thus at any given time, support by autistics ebbs and flows, alliances shift.

If people who are diagnosed, misdiagnosed, self-diagnosed, in the process of getting a diagnosis, seeking a diagnosis, or wannabees have an agenda, the degree to which they will push that agenda, and the lengths they will go to varies. Some are fine with fostering discussions, creating think tanks, signing petitions, initiating letter writing campaigns, etc. Others will infiltrate organizations, rise to board membership level, and then attempt to destroy those organizations. Still others will engage in online trolling or offline harassment, using covert and overt methods. They may do things to their target like:

- Crank call them at home
- Crank call them at work
- Vandalize their cars and homes
- File false police reports against them
- Make false reports to child protective services organizations
- Make false allegations against people to their employers
- Steal their identities
- Steal their online accounts
- Troll them
- File false reports with social media sites for violation of services
- Etc.

People who are diagnosed, misdiagnosed, self-diagnosed, in the process of getting a diagnosis, seeking a diagnosis, or are wannabees, can sometimes find themselves targeted if they fail to involve themselves in the schemes of the more militant people and factions. In addition to all of this, there are individuals that are deemed to be very important leaders for each particular faction. To follow one person may automatically mean you become the enemy of many different factions.

There are of course people who do not have autism that circulate in the online and offline autism world. These may be:

- Parents
- Relatives
- Friends
- Teachers
- Doctors
- Researchers
- Curiosity seekers
- People with an agenda such as
-Quacks who are looking to sell something
-Scam artists who are looking to make money

And they may be

- ☐ Vaxers
- ☐ Anti-vaxers
- ☐ Pro-cure
- ☐ Anti-cure
- ☐ Proponents of quack therapies
- ☐ Proponents of conspiracy theories

There are many more factions than the ones I have listed here. But what it really boils down to is that many of these people, no matter what faction they belong to, are interested in self-promotion first, being right –or being seen as being right-second, and helping people third. It should be noted that "self-promotion" in this context can mean promotion of their cause in addition to promoting themselves. Many of these people feel that if you go against their cause, you go against them personally.

Keeping all this in mind, you should remember that any one of them may be the person you are buying a book from. Each of them knows that if they think they *can* brainwash you into believing in them or in their cause, they *will*, and if this means lying to you, so be it.

What you will find out about some of the most militant "activists" if you go deep into the forum threads, chat-rooms and conversations, or if you have private correspondence with them, is the truth. Many of these people were bullied when they were children. They were often disciplined by their parents and relatives. They were fired from their jobs. They have criminal records.

Through the illustrious and ubiquitous internet, however, they have been given a voice, and if they can crowd their way into a conversation, or shout from the electronic hilltops, they will.

If they can write a book, all the better.

I have observed that people like this –who are mostly just social misfits, or else people with behavioral problems –are learners. They have been told most of their lives by bullies and earnest people alike what is "wrong" with them, and they have memorized what things are "the right things to do." Hiding behind their computer screens, they only show the "good" and "right" side of themselves and not the "bad" and "wrong."

They may have multiple user names with multiple accounts set up under each of them. They may have pay pal buttons set up under each of those accounts to collect money for many different causes. They may be on the government dole. They may have poor work histories and criminal records.

But they don't let you know about any of that.

Instead, when they become well-known enough on the web, they publish a book. All their friends buy it despite the fact that clinically speaking, what they have written may be bunk at best, and may be dangerous at worst.

And then they go on tour.

Reality Number Eight: Autism Conventions don't have your best interest in their hearts either. Neither do the "authors" that speak at them.

For the people who organize these conventions, it's all about the money. Elyse Bruce and I know someone who was diagnosed autistic who was asked year after year to present his work at a convention. The problem was that the people who organized and operated this convention never bothered to ask if this person was diagnosed autistic. Billed as an autistic, they didn't seem to care whether or not the person was diagnosed. They simply assumed he was.

But he was indeed a good draw for them. Lots of people came to see him, and bought many of the products he had for sale.

So it is with authors.

If a convention promoter says "Autistic author So-And-So will be speaking at…" be sure to find out for yourself whether or not the author in question is actually diagnosed. And even if the author is what he or she purports to be, ask yourself why they are there and whether or not they are really going to give you what you came to get.

If you have someone in your life who is autistic, you see them everyday. Their story is very remarkable. Why are you paying good money to read or listen to someone else's story? Why are you paying to read their book? If you have an answer to either or both of those questions, then going to see such an author might be worth it. If you cannot answer one or both of those questions, then why are you going to see them?

Reality Number Nine: Just because a book is published doesn't mean it's published.

When I state this reality, I am not making reference to self-publishing. Self-publishing is a form of publishing as valid as any other. I have done it many times. The book you are reading now is self-published.

But it is important for purchasers of books in particular to understand what they are buying, whether they buy that book in a store, order it from an online marketplace, or buy directly from the publisher.

For one thing, in the traditional publishing world the degree to which an item is published depends on how you define publishing. There are publishers, for example, who do nothing but publish books about autism.

Keep in mind when researchers publish something in medical journals, these journals examine the research before allowing the research to be published. This is not necessarily true with material about autism that gets published outside of that realm.

Generally, in a time when print is dying, publishers these days may look at a book from three different vantage points:

1. Is the book going to be something that people will want to read?
2. Is the book something that will sell?
3. Is the book something that's not going make the publisher legally liable to someone in some way?

A book can be an utter waste of paper, but if it meets the above criteria, it may be published, especially by publishers who only publish literature about autism.

Journals that are autism specific may operate the same way, as do many autism charities and autism organizations which publish newsletters.

Reality Number Ten: Sometimes the book you're buying isn't the book you're buying.

A popular children's book about a child with Asperger Syndrome actually has nothing to do with Asperger Syndrome specifically. It was purely incidental that the main character had AS. The author has admitted this fact in author interviews.

In early editions, which did not sell remarkably well, the autistic character was not promoted by the publisher. Once the publisher began promoting the autistic character is subsequent editions, however, the book sold better.

That's something to think about in you are a consumer.

Some Final Words on These Realities:

In a day when a few clicks of a computer mouse can buy a book, you have never been a more powerful consumer than you are now. As a consumer, you have in within your power to determine which books stay on the market and which don't. Further, you have it within your power to determine which "autistic" authors make a career out of their supposed autism and which don't.

Many people who claim to be autistic authors don't actually have autism. Whether an author is autistic or not, many cannot be trusted. Their dispersal of information about autism is seldom altruistic. Often times "autistic superstars" are the worst offenders.

Don't be fooled by them.

The Appearance of Autistics in Literature

Now that we come this far, I'd like to take a moment to talk about autistics as they *appear* in literature, and then I will return to a commentary on autistic authors.

On the online autism social media sites, I've often seen it written that the media ought to have more autistic characters in their TV shows. I've also heard it mentioned that beyond the scope of storybooks there ought to be more books that have autistic characters in them.

Hmm.

While I agree that these thoughts may be relevant, I have to ask myself what "autistic" looks like, and to what degree it should be represented. Additionally, having just spent a few thousand words asserting that there are diagnosed, misdiagnosed, and self-diagnosed autistics who cannot be trusted as authors, can I say that somebody who isn't autistic can be trusted to portray autism accurately?

In regards to the depiction of autism, do we take the DSM IV, DSM V, or ICD-10 and craft a character around the descriptors housed within those publications? Do we watch *Rainman* or *Mozart and the Whale* and write a book that imitates what we see? Do we go to an autistic meet-up group and ask the people there for their opinions? Do we visit an online forum where autistics and self-diagnosed autistics snipe back at forth at one another and take one of *them* to use as our character?

The answer to all of those questions ought to be "no."

While it is true that autistics ought to be represented in literature as realistically as possible, there is no one representation that can be made. If you have seen one autistic, you have seen one autistic. Therefore, you cannot draw an autistic character and expect that that character will be representative of the autistic population as a whole. What you *can* do, however, is draw on the behaviors of people who have a bonafide and provable diagnosis and go from there. Reading research and reviewing studies on autism also helps.

I have done this in a *general* way in two of my books. "Geo-213: The Lost Expedition" (a novel) and "Geo-213: The Lost Stories" (a book of four short stories) has a main character on the spectrum, although I do not say this outright in the books. There are two reasons for not revealing that at least one of my characters is autistic:

1. I knew when I wrote both books that the DSM V would be coming out before their publication, and there was a likelihood that Asperger Syndrome and

other autism delineations would be stricken from the list of autism spectrum disorders, and

2. I wanted to see if my readers would be able to identify a character as "autistic" if I didn't label the character as such.

I am aware that some Aspies have read the books, and to date, no one has come forward and said which character it is they believe to be on the spectrum. Further, no one has come forward with even a suspicion that any of my Geo-213 characters might be on the spectrum.

The cat was let out of the bag when I posted a blog article on the MIC blog. Harren Trober is on the spectrum. Where he lies on the spectrum is something I am *still* leaving open deliberately.

Thus far, there have been no objections to Harren's character being autistic.

Interestingly, some of those people who have read the book see Harren as neurotypical or "normal." They hold this view because he supposedly holds the traits neurotypical or normal people are stereotypically thought to have. He's well-educated, gainfully employed, married, he gets along fairly well with his coworkers most of the time, has a diverse range of interests (although he perseverates on just a few) is multi-talented, has the ability to adapt to crisis situations, but is somewhat socially inept.

Sometimes, he gets into verbal or physical altercations with his closest friends and colleagues, and he has a poor working relationship with his boss, but this does not happen often.

How do these qualities make him autistic?

Well, this is what my real life autistic friends are like, much to the chagrin of those online diagnosed, misdiagnosed, and self-diagnosed autistics who have a laundry list of supposed symptoms.

Many autistics that I have either met socially, or whom I know personally, do things like teach college, run companies, write books, care for children, etc. Seldom in real life have I ever fallen witness to any of the types of meltdowns or lapses of judgment we so often see supposed autistics make online. In fact, only once have I seen an example of a meltdown, and that was an autistic woman rocking underneath a table. She was at an autism convention. The duration of the rocking was very short, and after she was finished, she gave a lecture in front of over two hundred people that lasted some twenty minutes.

As a writer, I am writing from experience, and so Harren Trober reflects the experiences I have observed.

This is not to say that autistics do not act like any of the ones we see on TV or the big screen. I am very aware that there is a spectrum of autistics, and there is a spectrum of affectations. For as many people on the spectrum that I personally know who are leading productive lives, there are many that I don't know who are so affected by autism as to be institutionalized.

Well, in the interest of full disclosure, I do know one person who is severely affected whom I see almost every day. I've never heard him speak. He goes to a special school by day and lives with his mother by night. Much of the time I have known him, he stands with his hands up by his shoulders. They shake, tremble, and flap constantly. Yet he smiles when I say hello to him, and he seems to enjoy it when he, myself, and his mother, are in good humor.

What I am told from *most* from people I meet is that I should craft a *good* autistic character for my books and stories. One who is capable. One who actually accomplishes something for a living. One who doesn't have any significant marital problems or big interpersonal relationship quandaries going on. But the biggest source of criticism that I get comes from those who *hate* such well-mannered successful autistic people. For this latter group, when I write a character like this, it means I have supposedly set a bar for them which they believe they are incapable of attaining.

These people are often ones who defend autistic criminals, often blaming the stifling "system" for "causing an autistic to go bad." Or they believe that autistics are incapable of functioning in schools designed primarily by and for "neurotypicals."

In my defense I would like to say that whenever I place an autistic character into a book, I do so with considerable deliberation, discretion, and care. Characters are portrayed not only according to what I have witnessed, but what I have learned through reviewing research and studies.

When going through teacher training a long time back, I had the benefit of teaching learning disabled and special education students in many different schools. I asked the special education teachers back then what the diagnoses were of the kids I would be working with.

A typical reply was usually:

> "Oh, that one's been diagnosed by the school psychologist with ADHD. That one has Asperger Syndrome. That one has NVLD. That one has OCD and Anxiety disorder. But you can't go by a school psychologist's diagnoses. We just label them with something so we can get the state funds to educate them they way they need to. Most of these kids are either slow learners, or kids with behavioral problems which can be conveniently pigeonholed into something in the DSM. But remember, there are five or six different diagnoses in the DSM that could fit each and every one of them, and only a rigorous diagnostic analysis could find the diagnosis that is right for them."

And so the lesson I learned that day: In terms of people who claim they have a diagnosis, what you see is seldom what you get. Ergo I can only base my characters on autistic individuals whom have *proven* to me that they have been diagnosed, and/or base my characters on what I've read in research and studies.

Regrettably or fortunately, depending on your point of view, I seldom see real life autistics trading barbs with people as they do online and I do *not* see them conniving behind each other's backs. I do *not* see them ganging up on others and picking on people until their victims are near suicidal. The real life autistics that I know are mostly employed in good jobs, are financially solvent, or have little debt, are involved in friendships and amorous relationships, are not prone to all the "deviant" sexual proclivities described by many of those misdiagnosed and self-diagnosed people in the online forums, are upstanding citizens, do not have a criminal record, and have saved for their retirement.

Then again, I know mostly high-functioning autistics.

But, to be succinct, you will find no autistics portrayed as loud-mouthed driveling semi-lunatics in my books. I am told by real autistics that this is admirable, but have been lambasted by online "autistics" for not deliberately stupefying my autistic characters.

So be it.

My pen will continue to write for as long as I am able, and for as long as readers wish to read what I have written.

Before proceeding to talk about a few other autistic characters I've written into my books, I am going to take my virtual newspaper and THWACK Stephen King on the nose for his portrayal of an autistic character in his novel The Regulators. Fans of King should understand that my motive is not to impugn King or his writing. I happen to own quite a few books of his, and enjoy re-reading many of them many times over. Salem's Lot, Bag of Bones, and The Stand happen to be three of my favorites. IT is particularly notable for its depiction of the pains of childhood.

But whereas King may be a literary genius when writing about children and childhood, I think he falls short when trying to depict people with certain kinds of mental illness. I could pick through everything of his that I've read in an attempt to weed out the characters I'm thinking of, but won't. We're talking about autism here.

Writing as Richard Bachman, King, in The Regulators, sets his characters in the middle of the Midwest. When an autistic boy (Seth) becomes possessed by a demon, the demon uses the boy's expansive and creative mind to move imagination into reality.

The solution to the problem from the many different characters' perspective is to kill Seth, but the boy has his own solution: He must delve deeper into the recesses of his own mind and lock out the demon from the portions of his brain which the demon uses to create evil. Once that's done, he, or he and one or more of the other characters, can go on the offensive.

Fine. Except predictably, for most of the story, Seth is literally a drooling idiot (and I am not using that term to be mean, his behavior literally fits the definition of the words. He drools, and he behaves in a manner that can be called idiotic), and not only that, but a *complaint* drooling idiot, who apart from minor toileting deficiencies, is not much of a problem whatsoever to his caretakers when life is normal. In other words, King/Bachman implies that an autistic individual who has little or no presence of mind outwardly, may be sane inside his or her head and knows (on the inside) not only know what is going on in the real world, but can control the degree to which he or she interacts with it.

To the autistic boy in <u>The Regulators</u>, his mind is a cave, and he can run through it, shutting doors to private places, and opening doors to places he wants his enemies to see.

What a wonderful fantasy!

If only this were true!

But unfortunately, as much as people would like to believe any one of a number of theories about what autism looks like from the inside out, no one can give in to any one theory because science has yet to figure out a way to inhabit the autistic mind and look out onto the world from inside of it.

Seth also has three traits autistic people are thought by many not to have: Empathy, a sense of awareness, and the ability to understand what others are thinking. To back up my assertion, I offer these three points as evidence:

1. He seems to understand how much his caretaker hurts as the result of the demon's activities.
2. He is aware that he is possessed.
3. He understands that the demon hates Seth's bowel habits so much that it vacates his body while he's on the pot.

We understand these things once we get inside Seth's mind.

In all fairness, I believe autistics are very empathetic, have a good sense of awareness, and do have an ability to understand what others are thinking. I have seen these traits displayed in abundance in people on the spectrum. But given that the DSM IV cites a lack of empathy as being a symptom of autism, King's inclusion of Seth's empathetic nature in his book is not true to medical science even if it is true to life.

What makes the book worse is the way the boy's caretaker (who is *not* his mother) sees him. She has adopted her dead brother's child, and she and her husband have tried to continue raising him. She describes him as strange, sometimes a nuisance, inconvenient, but nearly always in a loveable way. This pathos seems to me to seem unrealistic given what I know of how mothers, fathers, and caretakers feel about their autistic charges. Yes, there is love, and yes, they can see the autistics they care for as lovable. But as much as there may be love, there is also a range of emotions that any caretaker would associate with a child. More, in fact, because autistic children can be very difficult to raise.

Emotions I would have liked to see Seth's caretaker express are angst, fear, anger, hate rage, sadness, sorrow, depression, and others. Seth's adoptive mother displays these emotions...but only against the demon that has taken Seth over.

Still, we must give King points for making the attempt to portray autism as realistically as he knows how. But I would have expected more from him considering that Seth's character is the pin around which the whole novel revolves.

My point in writing this is that if writers do not understand autism, it's best not to write an autistic character into their cannon, especially when the plot of the piece they're writing depends on something the autistic character does.

The quality of King's lifelong work reads like a heartbeat. He has works that rate on the upside and others that fall below the line. For me, The Regulators is one of the pieces that don't make the grade, in my opinion, because of Seth's poorly drawn character. It's the one disappointing facet of an otherwise glowing gem of a book.

I should say however, that as an author, I know that there have been many times when I have attempted to write about something and have failed miserably. We cannot be 100% perfect, and even if we write something that wins a prize or an award, (as King and I both have -and he more times that I), it is unreasonable to expect that we can consistently write that well.

As a side note, it should be stated that King makes a similar attempt to make a special needs individual a hero in his Dreamcatcher novel, but I think he also fails there. In that example, the character in question is not autistic, but has Down Syndrome, if memory serves.

And so in future, Mr. King, in my opinion, would do well to do a little more research into the diagnosis he is trying to write about. He should find people who have the diagnoses and get to know them. Only after doing that should he write. As much as it is nice to see an autistic character shown as a hero in one of his books, since his character isn't exactly autistic in the diagnosable sense of the word --or in terms of how his character's mind operates-- one could almost say that there is no autistic hero in his book at all.

In short, his autistic character in The Regulators is about as believable as an Indian portrayed by Rock Hudson in the movie *Winchester 73*.

And now I must chastise those in the autism community who think the autistic character in The Regulators is the greatest thing since sliced bread. Yes, he's very heroic and all of that, and we would certainly love to see real world autistics be just as heroic. But many times we read stories in the newspaper of people on the spectrum doing heroic things, so let's stick with them for our role models, shall we? Or else let's chose to read fictional literature more befitting of the diagnosis.

I have mentioned that I portray autistics in the literature I publish as I see them. When I make them hard working, earnest individuals who are religious, philanthropic, and happily involved in healthy monogamous relationships with lovers and spouses, I am basing these characters on autistics whom I personally know. When my friends on the spectrum see such characters in print, I get compliments.

Online "autistics" are much more critical.

To combat this criticism, one of the things my real world friends on the spectrum have suggested is that I write a book in which autistics on the net are represented "exactly" as they are."

Aside from the fact that autism presents itself differently in each person who is diagnosed with it, I cannot in good conscience write a book about autistics "exactly" as they are because, thanks to misdiagnosed, self-diagnosed, and wannabe "autistics" intermixing with the diagnosed autistic population, it has become almost impossible to discern what is "autistic" and what isn't.

I also get a lot of flack from online posers when I write about issues true to the heart of the autistics I know. One autism advocacy organization -which is staffed primarily with people who admit privately that they are not autistic- has advocated for a "national autism registry." No autistic that I personally know wants this registry. They have fears of being tracked, fears of being unwitting test subjects in covert experiments, fears of being discriminated against as their label follows them everywhere.

So I wrote a blog article on this topic.

The stream of vituperation that came in from online posers is something I cannot even begin to describe, but the support I got from people who actually have diagnoses was equally immense.

Writing those articles reinforced for me exactly how much misdiagnosed, self-diagnosed, and wannabe autistics are messing things up for diagnosed autistics.

Evil Creeps In: A Tale of Exorcism required me to read up extensively on what the Holy Roman Catholic Church had to say about exorcism, and I had to research what the Lutheran Church Missouri Synod's perspective was on the topic as well. For my characters --who were both well-educated theologically-- to sound like they knew what they were talking about, I had to study both the Catholic and Lutheran catechisms as well as Catholic and Protestant Bibles. (I have read many different versions on the Protestant Bible cover to cover many times for spiritual guidance and in preparation for things I planned to write which had religion as an underpinning to the main story. But for Evil Creeps In, a re-read seemed necessary.)

Given the years of research this involved, one would think that I could easily apply the same effort elsewhere, and infiltrate the more nefarious, notorious and execrable areas of the net where supposed autistics and self-diagnosed autistics like to hang out.

I have done so to a degree.

In some cases, I have been a passive observer to the scheming and conniving that go on. In others, I have made a show of actively involving myself in their plans, but then bowing out on some pretense or other at the last moment. But it's interesting what you will find out when you are part of the "inner sanctum," so to speak. For one thing, once you are admitted into their confidence, what you will find out is that people claiming to be autistic on the net readily admit that they are not autistic and have never been diagnosed. In fact, privately, they characterize themselves as "social rejects" who fit in really well with autistics because "autistics are rejects too."

Pathetic as this may seem, it has its humorous side, because the autistics they believe they fit in with may not be professionally diagnosed either.

Another common element among these people is that they *do* have other diagnoses. Usually these are behavioral disorders. Specifically: conduct disorder, bipolar disorder, Operational Defiant Disorder. They may also have been diagnosed with schizophrenia, have learning impairments, and may be living with their parents. Many job hop, are unemployed, or have gotten into significant problems at work. Some have criminal convictions.

And so, no. I am not going to base my autistic characters on these people, because these people are liars and crooks with diagnoses and symptomologies that do not fall under the pervasive developmental disorder category in the DSM-IV.

For similar reasons, I am not inclined to seriously listen to any criticism from these pretend autistics for the way I portray real autistics in my books.

There was also one irony I encountered during my incognito sojourn into the grotty corners of the net, and that is that these supposed autistics, who were kind to me, Thomas Taylor, on Facebook and on similar social media sites, were the ones inciting the incognito me to work *against* Thomas Taylor.

Now, to a degree, these people can be fictitiously portrayed in literature. For an example, I would suggest reading

Elyse Bruce's marvelous novel <u>Glass On A Stick</u>. There you will at least see a realistic portrayal of self-diagnosed autistics, if not diagnosed autistics as well. What Bruce manages to accomplish in her book is to show how a group of these people can negatively affect one innocent person, or a group of well-meaning individuals.

I have also attempted to portray them in a short story of my own "The White Nurse."

We'll talk about "The White Nurse" and other literary publications next.

I've decided to use my own writing, as well as Elyse Bruce's, to illustrate my points. This is not because I believe my writing or hers to represent the apex of the type of literature that uses autism as subject matter, but because I believe the examples will best serve the purpose of making my points.

My points will come later. We will begin with *my* writing, but before we get into any lengthy discussion, it will be necessary to provide some context about the stories I am going to be introducing you to. There will be two of them to begin with.

The first is called "The White Nurse", and the second is called "Little Green Men." Both are ostensibly horror stories although "The White Nurse" is closer to a thriller than anything else, and "Little Green Men" borders on fantasy. They have been published in my 1115,000 world anthology <u>Ghostly Quintet: Five Tales of Ghosts, Apparitions, and the Beyond</u>. You shouldn't have to read the stories to understand what I am writing about here.

To begin with, it is important to understand that a work of fiction may have its roots in fact, but it is primarily a work of invention, imagination, fabrication, and fantasy. Still, this doesn't mean we can't have some realism intertwined with the make believe. In regards to horror, for example, whether or not a person believes in ghosts, goblins, demons, or what have you, we can still readily accept other, more real aspects of a story. If I use a place name, for example, like Chicago, and mention a few locations familiar to people who live in that city, those particular readers will have no problem believing the setting for the story actually exists.

As I have indicated, autism plays an important role in "The White Nurse" and "Little Green Men" and in those two stories, autism is the element that adds the touch of realism that was necessary to make the fictional aspects of the stories work.

"The White Nurse" is a story that has a man vs. man archetype as its subject. In this case, the warring parties are autistic advocates and anti-vaccine proponents, with an actual autistic person, "Michael" playing the role of hero, although he doesn't actually come into the conflict until the very end.

Without spoiling the plot too much, I will say that both sides are at each other's throats throughout the story, with one side going to extremes –murder, specifically- in order to vanquish the opposite side.

In this particular story, I could have used any type of conflict to lead the reader to the finale. Keeping this in mind, it is arguable that autistic factional politics are incidental to the story. Given that most mills are capable of grinding any grist that's fed into them, why choose autistic politics for my story?

Well, I do have an ulterior motive for writing my horror books, and that is to explore evil a little. Specifically in keeping with the purposes set forth in the Author's Note and Afterword of Evil Creeps In: A Tale of Exorcism, I was attempting to glorify God, impart morals, show what's good and what isn't, and elucidate the difference between Holy and evil. Additionally, in Ghostly Quintet I was trying to show the consequences that ensue when someone *seeks out* evil, and secondly, I was trying to show how mental illness or mental differences can positively or negatively impact one's interaction with evil.

In "The White Nurse", we see the negative side of how mental illnesses and mental differences affect the characters' responses to and interactions with evil, and in "Little Green Men" –a story where the protagonist, who has Asperger Syndrome, vanquishes "aliens"- we see the positive side.

As I have said in the Afterword of Ghostly Quintet, there is hardly a way that I can talk about mental illness without getting taken to task by someone. And as I have indicated in the Author's Note of Ghostly Quintet, nothing I have written in the book is meant to offend, yet I felt that writing about mental illness and mental differences in story format was an important thing for me to do. Mental illness exists. Mental differences exist. They are real. There is a statistical possibility that someone we know is affected by a diagnosis, and there could be times in our own lives when we find ourselves diagnosed with something, be it as transient as an extended but finite period of depression, to something much more impacting.

Yet regardless of what kind of diagnosis someone has, the world turns, and we all must find our own way to at least exist on it. Some people are more successful than others. The question is, when it is possible to exercise some degree of control over whatever ails us, how much control will we choose to exercise?

With each of these stories, you can just as easily subtract the characters' diagnoses out of the equation and you ought to be able to see that it is the characters at their core who make the decisions which get them into trouble. And that is my point in writing the stories I am talking about here.

While I know it isn't true in all circumstances, I'd like to think that much of the press we see which vilifies people with mental illness is just plain wrong. When we see a shooting, oftentimes, we read something like "The shooter, who had Asperger Syndrome..." but how often do we read "The shooter, who had no diagnosis whatsoever...?" There are plenty of diagnoses listed in the forthcoming DSM V, and it seems like the press trots them out whenever a particularly heinous crime is committed. And where there is no data as to whether or not a perpetrator of a crime has a diagnosis or not, the press implies that one exists.

To go on a brief tangent, why does the press vilify people with diagnoses, and only *certain* diagnoses at that? What would happen if the press stated, "The shooter, who had diabetes..." or "The shooter, who had celiac disease..." It seems neither the press or the general public have a problem with autistics being blasted in print when a crime is committed, but how would the public feel if it was written that" The shooter, who was black..." or "The shooter, who was homosexual..." or "The shooter who was sexually molested in their childhood...?"

The fact is, plenty of people do terrible things for reasons that cannot be attributed to a diagnosis, but one thing that is interesting to note is that people are more likely to look at a particular action or deed and say "that's wrong," when a person *does* have a diagnosis. So what I want the reader to do with the stories I have written, is to think about the stories in terms of how my bad acting characters would stand up to moral, ethical, and spiritual standards if their diagnoses were removed from the equation. Could anyone take away their diagnoses and say that what they are doing is *good*? If so, then a person who makes that pronouncement is prejudiced against people with a diagnosis. If not, then he or she is more willing to forgive "normal" people than those with a diagnosis when they do evil things.

My stories seem to differ from many of the other stories and books out there which have autistic characters as protagonists. To me, it is not quite correct to continually throw "autistic as hero" at the reader all the time and expect it to stick. While we would all like to see people with disabilities portrayed in a good light, we must also recognize the fact that, like people without diagnoses, people *with* diagnoses act with motive, not just motivation.

And this, I believe, is the central fault with most literature which has an autistic as the hero: There is no real explanation as to why the autistic behaves in a heroic manner.

People will argue that nobody needs a motive to be a hero, but these people should ask themselves how willing they would be to take a bullet for someone else, or rush into a burning building and rescue someone. Our heroes in law enforcement and the fire department put themselves in harm's way everyday, but these people are special. Not only are they trained to do these things, but they have prepared their minds for the possibility that they will need to act heroically. If you were walking down the street and found yourself having to act on the spur of the moment, could you do what those people do?

In regards to most literature I've read where an autistic person is the hero, the fault, then, is that the autistic acts like a robot, either without thought, or, if there is any thought involved, hackneyed, stereotypical thought. Usually, when the moment to act arrives, the autistic person rises above himself or herself and does what is required to remedy the problem, and sometimes, the action is entirely out of character, and usually outside the bounds and limits of autism too. As readers, we are supposed to be inspired by this sort of tripe, and perhaps hope that if a fictional autistic character can excel beyond the limits of their diagnoses, real autistic people can do it too.

For me personally, if I am going to have an autistic be a hero and act heroically, I will have them do so *within* the bounds of their diagnoses. In this way, I can show how fictional autistics, just by being themselves, have the potential to be heroes, and cause the reader to understand that it may be quite possible for *real* autistics in the *real* world to be heroes too.

But if autistics can be heroes, they can also be villains. If I am going to be honest to my readers, I must have autistic characters who act with evil intent.

To date, I have not tackled that particular challenge, opting instead to have autistic wannabees and self-diagnosed autistics be the villains.

Never have I portrayed self-diagnosed autistics as villains more blatantly than in "The White Nurse." "The White Nurse" gives us an opportunity to judge behaviors, because the characters in that story engage in many behaviors that we can easily judge.

Ironically, in the anti-vaxer Barbara's case, her behaviors are almost always driven by paranoia and irrational fears, and are arguably excusable for that reason. But she seeks out trouble when she chooses to attend the evil autism advocate's (Jonquil's) lecture at an autism convention.

In fact, if Jonquil is evil, we can say that Barbara is seeking out evil when she elects to sit down and listen to Jonquil's speech. We can excuse Barbara's reactions to the subsequent adversity, but we cannot so easily excuse her actions that ultimately lead to the adversity she experiences.

"The White Nurse" was a difficult story to write. After reading multiple peer-reviewed studies by qualified medical researchers, my opinion is that autism is genetic in origin. I know that there are many unproven theories about the causes of autism, and I know that vaccines as the culprit is tops on that list of unproven theories. People who have read "The White Nurse" may believe I was trying to make fun of anti-vaxers. This was not the case. While technically it is Barbara's autistic son Michael who is the hero of the story, Barbara is also a hero when one considers the vital role she plays in bringing the self-diagnosed/wannabee criminals to justice.

Hopefully, readers of that story will understand how my attempts to address a familiar topic (subterfuge in the war between pro-vaxers and anti-vaxers) required me to honestly reflect in writing my feeling that it is anti-vaxers who come out of it taking the biggest berating, the biggest beating, and the biggest bullying, from their opposition. Despite the fact that I disagree with the idea that vaccines cause autism, I must accept that though anti-vaxers are very fervent about arguing their points, pro-vaxers, in my opinion, tend to be the most unethical, underhanded, and aggressive when challenging the opposition.

If a writer is going to write about reality, they must translate or reflect that reality accurately for their readers.

How much control Barbara exercises over her desire to sink the opposition by hook or by crook should get an honorable mention too, because, as is the case with anti-vaxers, they do exercise considerable control when confronting the pro-vaxers. Yes, Barbara probably should have avoided Jonquil at the convention. Yet as a paying customer, it *was* Barbara's right to be there. It is reasonable, therefore, to expect that Barbara should gain admittance to the convention and attend without consequence. And so when Jonquil and her cronies view Barbara's attendance as an attack, and retaliate with disproportionate rage, the reader finds himself or herself admiring the restraint Barbara uses to deal with the situation.

I must acknowledge, however, that Barbara doesn't need to exercise too much control. I have given her a number of tools she can use which create an added buffer zone between her and her enemies. She has cameras, an alarm system, and phone taps. When you've got all that, you don't have to worry as much about attacks.

Still, Barbara's situation is atypical. A sticker on the door that says callers are under surveillance or that an alarm is present, is enough of a deterrent to make law abiding people think twice about paying a visit to whomever lives behind that door. But Jonquil & Company are at best persistent salespeople who ignore the No Soliciting sign and knock on the door, and are at worst violent criminals who will use any method they can to break in.

We don't know what quibble or squabble started the fight that ultimately wound up in near murder, but if the cause is partially attributable to mental illness, then both sides are technically at fault. While I am no pacifist, I think there are very few things in life worth going to war over, and if that's what Barbara and her enemies are doing, my opinion is that they should both give it up.

Likewise, I believe there are very few reasons to kill another human being. Self defense *might* be one reason, which is why I wouldn't have much of a problem if Michael killed the leader of the autism advocacy organization (Stoughton), but Stoughton, who is, in the end, the would be murderer, has inexcusable motives for killing.

I did quite a bit of research into the political factions of the autism world before I drafted *"The White Nurse."* I am sure I'm going to get criticism for the portrayal of some of the characters. However, it should be understood that the thrust of the story is that most of the "autistic" characters who behave badly in the story aren't actually diagnosed with autism. They only claim to be diagnosed. In fact, they may or may not have any one of many other diagnoses which could explain their manipulativeness and uncontrolled rage. What I was trying to show was that there are people out there who will use a diagnosis as a stepping stone to acquiring whatever it is they want from other people, and they will do so at the expense of people with a *real* diagnosis. I think this is a very nasty thing for people to do.

I have witnessed this phenomenon not just in the online and offline autism community, but in other disability communities as well. My feeling was that someone needed to write openly and honestly about this topic, and so it might as well be me.

To be succinct: My opinion is that when someone uses another person's diagnosis in order to get something from unsuspecting people, what they are really doing is stealing a diagnosis so that they can con other people for selfish and greedy purposes.

I doubt you will find that kind of deep thought put into most literature where autistics are major characters.

There are even deeper themes than this running through the story.

Barbara is not exempt from leveraging the particulars of a situation to her advantage. If her goal is to propel her theory that vaccines cause autism to the forefront, she is not above using manipulation to destroy the reputations of those who believe genetics are the cause.

No one in the story, except her son, Michael, comes out of the situation with their hands clean, although something else to consider is that if Barbara would have minded her own business, and/or if the "autism advocates" hadn't decided to push the envelope with her, Michael would never have had to "save" his mother by taking violent action against the murderous Stoughton. Through the plot of the story, I believe I have demonstrated the effect evil practiced in private can have on innocent people.

To an extent, Michael is a Christ figure. He literally risks death in order to save his mother, and through his actions, he gives Stoughton a just warning about what happens when a self-serving, exploitative and predatory individual goes on the offensive to the bitter end. The sacrifice he makes is made freely, without thought, and with unconditional love for his mother.

When I wrote Michael's use of violence into the story, was this just a cheap shot to force some emotional reactions from my readers? Wouldn't it have been better if I had maybe just had Michael the autistic come into the room, yelling and screaming, and have Stoughton the poser come to a realization that what he was doing was wrong? Such a scene would have been akin to an autistic poser and imposter (Stoughton) facing the real autistic person (Michael). It would have made for very powerful reading.

However, my goal in the supernatural compilation was for my stories to have some basis in realism, and what I have seen time and time again is that those "autistic advocates" who aren't really diagnosed at all, will put autistics in the position of monkey in the middle, and they will do so with merciless disregard and outright indifference for the autistics they claim to advocate for. It seems to me that it is just and right to portray a fictional event in a manner that is true to life instead of in the hackneyed romanticized way so many other writers will often do.

I have seen people admit in private online forums that they do not have autism and were never suspected of having it, but in the more public online autism forums, they persist in claiming to have autism. These people will ruthlessly harass real autistics, going so far as to hijack their accounts, call up their places of business to sabotage their jobs, crank call them at home, file bogus complaints against them with the police department, and, if they meet in person, engage in physical altercations with them.

So if you didn't like how I wrote Stoughton's and Jonquil's characters, and if you found yourself hating how I concluded the story, recognize that characters very similar to the ones I have written about *could theoretically* exist for real, and events *could* happen that *could theoretically* be similar to the ones I describe in the story. I didn't have any people in mind when I designed my characters, nor did I have a particular situation in mind either, but both the characters and the situation represent a theoretical amalgam of some of the people and things I have seen.

But as we can see, the evil in this story is the evil that men and women do. No ghost or spirit from beyond the grave can be blamed for anything that happens in "The White Nurse."

For Barbara, the "ghost" she encounters may scare her, but scarier in my opinion is the lengths people are willing to go to in order to get what they want.

I will continue here by talking a little about my story, "Little Green Men" which can be found in my anthology Ghostly Quintet: Five Tales of Ghosts, Apparitions, and the Beyond.

It isn't necessary to read the anthology to understand what I am going to talk about here. All that is necessary is that you understand the main points I am trying to make. Point one was that many autistics in today's fiction seem to be stock autistics put in hackneyed heroic positions. My belief is that it is more realistic to portray autistics as themselves, where they may, in the course of their day to day activities, have occasion to act with heroism.

In "Little Green Men," Billy Meeks, a man with Asperger Syndrome, trusts Scott Trumble, a non-autistic, implicitly, and this is probably why the arguably devious Mr. Trumble doesn't try to deceive Billy for evil purposes. We know Billy has Asperger Syndrome, and this may be why Trumble doesn't take advantage of him, but one question comes to mind as we watch the two of them interact with one another: Can super intelligence be a mental illness and a liability?

It can certainly get them into trouble. Trumble winds up on the radar of foreign spies and eventually gets kidnapped by "little green men." Both the characters find themselves implanted with "alien" chips.

Neither character is doing anything sinful per se, but they are both seeking knowledge that it is best for them not to have. What they experience when the abduction takes place is their just desserts for dabbling in things that are none of their business. Before they began their quest for knowledge, life was the closest thing to Eden for them. Once they crossed the line, their lives became a kind of living hell.

The story seems very simple and straightforward, and it's an easy read. With a little polishing, it could be a boy's adventure yarn, but there is another aspect of the tale that I think most people might not see unless I pointed it out to them, and that would have to do with the little green men.

The little green men are little more than marionettes, with people we cannot see (until the very end) pulling the strings. The goal of the puppeteers is to use the green men to spy and to do their dirty work for them. Not a very nice thing to do, but at least it is the green men being manipulated, and not people. Trumble, on the other hand, has his own spy network. The people who send information to a newsletter he puts out are doing it of their own free will, but by publishing his newsletter, and by offering a select and lucky few the occasional byline, Trumble gives these pawns reason to continue subscribing to his game. They are essentially Trumble's little green men. Interestingly, Trumble shows about as much lack of caring toward most of these living people as the real spies do about their little green men.

By the end of the story, Billy becomes a little green man, following Trumble's instructions to the letter without stopping to think about whether what he is being told to do is right or wrong. He trusts that Trumble's motives are correct and honorable.

And here is where we have another accurate portrayal of an autistic in literature: The autistic as victim.

You can see here that in "Little Green Men" I have steered clear of the familiar story of an autistic being bullied. That sort of pathos, while useful in a public service announcement kind of way, is old hat and, in my opinion, amateurish. What's needed, in my opinion, is to show ways in which autistics get taken advantage of, because this is something that happens every day.

I even make the story difficult for readers to some degree.

While we can say, for example, that Trumble has given Billy a choice about joining him in his conspiracy theory ventures, Billy really has no choice. In looking at the way Billy's mind works, we can see that Billy lives moment to moment, and goes through life jumping from task to task. (And the story reads choppy and chaotic to reinforce that concept.) Having been tempted by his perseverative interest -UFOs, Billy has very little compulsion *not* to follow Trumble's lead.

At the end of the story, I give the reader no clue as to whether or not Billy leaves Mr. Trumble, and goes to college (which is what his parents believe he should be doing). Instead, I leave it open. What do you think Billy will do in light of all that has happened? And if he elects to continue working alongside of Trumble, where do you suppose he will wind up?

Trumble's activities, as well as those of the activities of the spies, should give us pause two ask ourselves four questions: How much are we are manipulated by others? How much do we manipulate others? How do other people manipulate us? And how do we manipulate others?

The subtle way in which Trumble manipulates people exemplifies how evil manipulates us without us knowing it. Little do thousands of people know that by sending letters to

Trumble's newsletter, they are providing him with the information he needs to track a spy network of little green men. Could it be that *you* are being misled in some subtle way? And what will be the ensuing consequences if the person or entity manipulating you turns out to be doing it for evil purposes?

Given the themes I was exploring in Ghostly Quintet, I think people will have an appreciation for the fact that I have put autistic characters in such prominent and heroic places in them.

Ghostly Quintet is arguably the most controversial book I have published thus far given its content and themes, however, one moral I have neglected to point out until now is that everyone who sins, regardless of how egregious those sins are, may be forgiven, either by God or by the people who have been sinned against or by both. This is made clear in the Bible, and applies whether we believe in God or not. When people do terrible things, they are usually capable of choosing to repent, to reform, and to embark in a new direction, and when they ask for forgiveness, we should motivate ourselves to forgive. The Bible tells us that God forgives all the time. We should follow His lead. We should even forgive if He deems a sin unforgivable, and recognize that refusing to forgive a sin is ultimately His decision to make and not ours.

While this is a preachy moral to insert anywhere, my purpose in pointing it out in this book is to further elucidate that this moral could not be so easily seen without the autistic characters I have written into Ghostly Quintet.

In Elyse Bruce's novel, Glass On A Stick, we see a theme similar to the one I have written about in "The White Nurse," but, whereas my short story is rooted in horror, Elyse's novel is a mainstream "fictional story inspired by true events."

In "The White Nurse," we have two opposing camps fighting one another, with a supposed supernatural sub-plot thrown in for good measure. In Elyse's book, we have two opposing camps involved in an online and offline fracas without any supernatural elements to obscure the essence of what is taking place. I think we can agree that many times, when a writer removes fantasy and the fantastical from fiction, what remains can be horrific in its implications. To state this point differently, if I have served up a garnished and embellished meal to my readers, and given it to them with entertainment, Elyse gives our meal to us raw.

Which is more horrific?

Elyse's is, in my opinion, because everything is laid out plain and simple, so we can get a good look at it. Whereas some restaurants have décor and circuses to go with their meals, most of us like to see what we're eating without distraction. What Elyse nakedly shows us about self-diagnosed autistics and autistic wannabee posers is not particularly palatable.

"The White Nurse" is a short story. Given its form, it is not designed to provide lengthy details about the machinations which take place *before* the culminating events that happen as we read. The reader must make inferences and draw conclusions. But in Glass On A Stick, time and time again, we see into the heads of the important characters, and are made to share in the madness of those who perform the most dastardly deeds.

This is how the two pieces of work can cover essentially the same theme but each be relevant independently or juxtaposed to each other. In fact, I would go so far as to say that if a reader of "The White Nurse" wants to get into the heads of any of the characters in that story, all they need do is read Glass On A Stick where they can pick a similar character and read pages upon pages of that character's thoughts.

And this brings me to another point with regard to the portrayal of autistics in literature: To make an autistic character believable, we need to get into their heads as much as we do the heads of characters who are *not* autistic. There is no better place to do this than in a novel, where space for this task abounds.

Emma Lynn and Carmel are the only two relevant characters who actually have autism in Glass On A Stick. Emma Lynn works for the "bad" side, and Carmel for the "good." But rather than have one character play the villain and the other character play the superhero, Bruce thankfully makes these characters more complex.

Like many autistics, Emma Lynn has fallen in with a group of people who accept her, and believes because this group treats her nicely, the members of the group must be nice. She begins to suspect something is wrong when the members of the group begin to do things to others that are not so nice. As the novel progresses, they turn on Emma Lynn, especially when she digs in her heels and refuses to do things which go against her moral sensibilities.

Carmel is a member of the "good" team. She is a high-functioning autistic "who needed a fair bit of time to formulate what she was going to say before actually speaking." What we see with the "good" group of people is that they make allowances for Carmel's differences, and accept her contributions at face value. In this way, we see that the "good" group thrives because everyone, whether they have disabilities or not, plays a part in the team's success, whereas on the "bad" team, both success and failure of the team can be attributed to the people with the biggest egos.

Bruce's portrayal of the ego in <u>Glass On A Stick</u> is almost a psychological study. Bruce will repeatedly put a character in a situation where no problem or crisis exists, and a character will invent a problem or crisis to use as an excuse for taking an action that is illegal, or immoral, or unethical, and most times completely unnecessary. Some of the pathways the villains walk to get to their final courses of action are ones that we see people walk in real life, and we will explore three of them a little bit here:

The "Bad Childhood" Excuse

We must admit that terrible things can happen in a person's childhood that will traumatize them and stay with them for life. However, I have noticed that much of the "trauma" *some* people claim to have gone through isn't trauma at all. It's just everyday real life experiences that are no different than those experienced by other people.

That some people are less able to cope with day to day existence is true, and we must be compassionate towards those people. But I'm not talking about those people particularly. I am talking instead about people who, due to no medical or personal motivation but selfishness, choose to be lazy, choose to be uneducated, choose to be jobless, choose to be rude or belligerent toward other people, choose to be unethical or immoral, choose to do things that are not law abiding, and...when their own behavior gets them into a jam...choose to act in a manner that will victimize other people.

Unless we have been locked in a cell all of our lives, we cannot help but see that the world at large follows certain laws and lives according to certain morals, values, and ethics. That the majority of the world's citizenry walks freely down the street and has not spent time in jail is a testament to the fact that these laws are not restrictive, that they are easily understood, and easily obeyed.

But they are apparently restrictive to some.

The same applies to morals, values, and ethics.

No matter who takes care of us after we are born, be it a parent or some case worker at an orphanage, our caretakers impart their morals, values, and ethics to us. Even if the intent of the caretaker is to be completely "neutral" about morals, values, and ethics, this neutrality in itself is something that will get picked up and incorporated into the mind of the person who is being cared for by virtue of being exposed to it. I believe this process persists, no matter what stage we are in life. Throughout life, our conscious selves behave like sponges, absorbing much of what we are exposed to.

The reciprocal event is to expel those morals, values, and ethics which we reject while retaining those which best fit our psyches.

It seems there is a segment of the population, however, that will argue that because of something they have suffered, be it a single traumatic event, or an entire childhood filled with traumatic events, they are entitled to shirk the laws, morals, values, and ethics that everyone else have, and live an existence that resembles anarchism.

Many times there is no traumatic event or traumatic childhood, and in reality, the "suffering" than a person claims to have experienced, was just and proper discipline for misbehavior. Perhaps the child was lazy, rude, defiant, etc., and all these things due to choice, not a diagnosis. Perhaps the child was repeatedly disciplined when the desired behavior was not demonstrated. One can see that years of this discipline could be interpreted by someone as being "abuse" but this interpretation is more indicative of a very insecure ego, one that doesn't want to admit that it's at fault.

While we can have sympathy for an insecure person like this, the world cannot stop turning for them. People like these are a liability to other people who have managed to get their ducks in a row. Tough as it is to have to say this, people are usually avoided, shunned, divorced, fired, fined, arrested, jailed, for a reason. If any of these things have happened, they have happened because the person doing the dumping or disciplining has not only identified an issue that needs to be addressed, but the issue is so overwhelmingly prevalent that they have felt compelled to act.

I have read cover to cover an e-book by a self-diagnosed person who claims victimhood throughout his life. An absent mother, and an incident of sexual abuse, I think, are clearly traumatic. But I have no sympathy at all for the excuses he makes for his subsequent behaviors. His father, being placed in the position of having to care for him and maintain a career, moves him from place to place around the country as opportunities present themselves, but the author runs away quite often, and for petty reasons. He doesn't like his father's girlfriend. He doesn't like the fact that he has to do work around the house. People in school don't understand him. He's jealous that his sister got to stay with his mother. Taking his chances, he prefers living on the street rather than living with the exact same kinds of problems and responsibilities that most other kids live with.

I find kids who struggled to live through such troubling times to be more inspirational than this author, who suggests that every negative event in his adult personal or professional life has its roots in his childhood. While other kids in his situation obey the law, go to school, do their chores, etc., this author writes about running away, hitchhiking, shoplifting, etc.

There is an incident where he is "on the road" and picked up by a man who hints at wanting sex, which the author refuses to provide. While the moment is very scary, I cannot help but think that the author put himself in harm's way by hitchhiking in the first place. Complicating matters further is that the author writes as though even as an adult, he should get sympathy from us, not only because of the trifling discipline he experienced as a child, but also because of this hitchhiking experience. To be honest, I have a hard time giving it to him, especially since he, as an adult, blames a lot of *current* events in his life for his failures.

As adults, we must at some point take responsibility for ourselves instead of making excuses. As much as the author I have just mentioned has indeed experienced traumatic events, I've read and heard of other people having far worse experiences, and who overcame their pasts to become very successful, and without help from anyone.

At any rate, the "I've had an abusive childhood, and that's why I should be allowed to skirt the law and act immorally and unethically now" argument is one Bruce explores in <u>Glass On A Stick</u>.

The "I'm Disabled" Excuse

If a person has a disability, it is understandable and proper that society should make allowances for that person. Making the life of a disabled person easier for them has the additional benefit of making life easier for those who are not disabled. If disabled people can care for themselves, people who aren't disabled can spend less time caring for them.

However, there are many self-diagnosed autistics, who have had a diagnosis of autism ruled out many times, who insist that they should receive special treatment due to their supposed "autism."

These people clamor for special treatment in school, jobs that they are not qualified to have out of school, and services they are not entitled to have. They may cite their "disability" as the reason for these perks, when in fact the only "disability" they may have is a poor attitude.

It is interesting to note how, one the one hand, people of this type will say that autism isn't a disability, but a difference, when they are fighting discrimination, but they will hypocritically cite their autism as a disability when trying to attain products and services they feel they are entitled to.

Perhaps for lazy people like these, it's the only way for them to get ahead. Having squandered their educations, and having failed to make it into college, having ruined their employment opportunities by willfully behaving in an antisocial manner, they now have no choice but to edge around and sneak ahead of people who have worked to get where they are, and edge around and sneak ahead of people with real disabilities, in order to survive.

I can remember what my teachers in elementary school used to tell us. "If someone asks to borrow a pen, or a pencil, or a piece of paper, or a ruler, don't give it to them. There are two reasons for doing this: When you grow up, no one is going to help you out when you need something. And you should never have to inconvenience yourself to help other people who are perfectly capable of helping themselves."

I and some of my classmates followed this rule. Others did not for fear of being "not liked" by their peers. Still others disobeyed the rule to deliberately sabotage their classmates. By encouraging their classmates to be ill-prepared, in other words, it increased the likelihood that the unpreparedness would hamstring them further on when it mattered. For instance, what if they were trying to get a job and the other candidate had forgotten a pen or a pencil, or even a resume? Maybe that would be all it took for that unprepared person to not get the job.

One of the ways many self-diagnosed people will try to convince themselves that what they are doing is right is to force other people to believe that they are handicapped, that they need a hand, and that, since they are denied that help now and were denied that help in the past, they are justified in taking unlawful, immoral, and unethical actions to get what they need. In reality, this group of people is no different than kids who forgot to bring a pencil to class.

Another attribute of people such as these is that what these people think they "need" is really just what they "want." Going back to that unnamed book I was talking about in the previous section, the author kept talking about needing to get out, needing to go away, etc. But as we read about his homelessness, and his trials and tribulations on the road, what we think is that what the author needed was to mind his father, study in school, do his chores, learn responsibility, learn how to manage money, learn how to accept his faults, and learn how to commit to a person, situation, or action.

As an adult, the author has had multiple marriages, multiple bad, unpaid debts, multiple jobs, multiple moves, some criminal convictions, and he still blames both his childhood and his undiagnosed "disability" for his problems.

Not to mention, bad fortune.

The "Bad Fortune" Excuse

This excuse is rooted in the sin of covetousness, and pertains to rank, position, and fame. It seems to me that when a person holds a position, or gets a promotion, or gets recognition that someone else wants, the someone doing the wanting gets jealous. While it often happens that good fortune is responsible for social and vocational success, oftentimes it is who you know, what you know, where you learned what you know, and how hard you work with who and what you know.

If a factory floor manager sees than one worker is more productive than another, that manager may give the better worker a compliment, a raise, or a promotion. If you or I see this, and aspire to get the benefits this other worker has gotten, chances are we will emulate the worker. We will adopt his attitude as our own, boost our quality to match his, boost our output to *beat* his, etc.

But if we are lazy, we will ascribe the recognition, raise, or promotion to favoritism, luck, or good fortune, and we will ascribe our own lack of success to the "fact" that the boss hates us, or the "fact" that the boss has unreasonable standards, or the "fact" that we have bad luck. Never mind that we cannot get into our boss's brain to know what he's thinking. Never mind that everyone else in the plant is subject to the exact same standards that we are, and that it is perfectly obvious that the praised and promoted fellow beat those standards. It couldn't possibly be that we are lazy, or that the quality of our craftsmanship is poor, or that our output is below target. It couldn't be that we have a poor attitude, a personality that is in some way lacking, etc.

We make all manner of excuses for ourselves when we don't want to admit that we have to work on bettering ourselves. But some people will take things in the wrong direction, and will try to acquire what other people have either by stealing it overtly or covertly, or by trying to convince others that they have been the victim of a string of bad luck.

We see Bruce's characters in <u>Glass On A Stick</u> use this kind of excuse to motivate themselves to misbehave, and I think we can freely admit that Bruce is not being unreasonable in having her characters behave this way. People do it all the time.

These three excuses or justifications for bad behavior are among the *many* Bruce explores in <u>Glass On A Stick</u>. The novel has additional value as well, because, what we are really doing by examining the excuses these self-diagnosed individuals make for themselves, is examining a whole segment of society that behaves this way: Those who are undiagnosed with autism (and who are sometimes undiagnosed with *anything*), but who choose to act immorally, unethically, and criminally.

The advantage to Bruce's novel, however, is that not only do we see a realistic portrayal of similar events that happens in real life, but we get into the heads of the self-diagnosed autistics involved in the scenarios. When we begin to see what they are thinking, and feel what they feel, it compels us much more than other fictional stories might.

Another area of contention in literature in my opinion is a "shallow" or poorly developed autistic character.

I am aware, for example, that there are people drawing comics in which autistic characters play the hero. This seems to me to be very insulting. Do autistics want their autism depicted as a kind of sidearm, weapon, or gimmick that they use to fight perceived injustices? And are the injustices perceived by the fictional superheroes ones that really exist in society, or are they just "injustices" in the jaded eyes of the comic book's author?

Even autistic autobiographies can be problematic in terms of how they depict autism or autistics. Although I have not read many autistic autobiographies, I believe that only two stand up to scrutiny and evaluation on the terms which I have described here. Tired are the familiar "You should admire me because I am autistic and have risen above my challenges" pieces of writing. And tired are the "I have been picked on all my life, because I'm autistic" claptrap. Another thing we no longer need to see is "Look at me! I'm autistic." It's been written. Insert the name of any other disability into this type of writing and you can see how it can be substandard (e.g. "Look at me! I have irritable bowel syndrome!")

Donna Williams and Temple Grandin are two authors I very much admire because both authors, in my view, see their autism as a facet of who they are. If anyone needs proof of that, all they need do is take a look at what Williams and Grandin are doing with their careers. Williams is a writer, painter, singer, and lecturer. Temple writes and lectures, but the primary focus of her career seems to center around animal handling. In her case especially, autism seems almost less an obstacle to her success than it was a personality trait which sometimes hindered her forward progress.

As we watch the movie about Temple Grandin (entitled <u>Temple Grandin</u> which was based on Grandin's book <u>Emergence</u>) we don't find ourselves pitying Grandin because she has autism, rather, we find ourselves admiring how she deftly circumvents the barriers thrown in her way by people who discriminate against her because she has autism.

So even though we are talking about autobiographies when we talk about Williams and Grandin, and not fiction, it is still worth stating that both Williams and Grandin make better heroes than autistics depicted fictionally in most of the literature that's out there.

I have striven to make any story in which autistics play a role better than anything else that is out there, and I believe Elyse Bruce has done the same.

Poor literature, in my opinion, is the kind where we are meant to pity people, or make fun of them, or root for them *because* they have a disability. Good literature, in my opinion, is the kind where we are meant to pity people, or make fun of them, or root for them because of their humanity or lack thereof. That such characters have a disability ought to be relevant to the story only in terms of how it limits a character's progress or contributes to a character's success. But how the character deals with those limitations or those extra added perks is what should be most important.

The other aspect of <u>Glass On A Stick</u> that we should examine is the book's portrayal of non-autistics and self-diagnosed autistics. Given that these characters are not autistic at all, one would think they are hardly worth mentioning, but because these people have managed to shove their way into the autistic population in the book, and characters similar to them have shoved their way into the autistic population for real, and because they have sometimes made a nuisance of themselves in the make believe world and people like them have done so in the real one, they should be looked at closely.

These characters can be seen as monkeys on the backs of autistics. They seem to be there no matter where autistics go. How difficult it must be for real autistics when a self-diagnosed autistic makes a pronouncement about autism that is utterly untrue that society winds up accepting as fact! How difficult it must be for real autistics when one of these posers commits a crime and the reputation of real diagnosed autistics are besmirched by it!

<u>Glass On A Stick</u> weaves together a tapestry of intrigues from the separate threads of little vendettas. When we see how it all comes together, we witness first hand how molehills become mountains, and we become impressed with how Bruce has hinted at how similar conflagrations come into being in the real world.

As we all know, not all autistic wannabees and posers are bad people who are detrimental to autistics. Many are well-mannered, good intentioned, philanthropic individuals who have attained high and admirable status in society. Yet the problem with those people is that they too, may be a liability to autistics. Do autistics want society to place unrealistic expectations on them because fakers and wannabees have demonstrated supposed successes?

If society at large is to understand autism, they need to see it up close and personal, and without distraction, skew, or bent. This is what Bruce attempts to do in the first place, and in the second place, she demonstrates how successful and unsuccessful self-diagnosed autistics and wannabees can be a liability to autistics.

We just don't see that in most autistic literature today or in literature that addresses autism.

I will now be discussing two of Elyse Bruce's published short stories "Flux in Time and the Batman Blacklist Boogie Band" and "The Incredible Realtor," both of which can be found in Elyse Bruce's anthology entitled <u>A Summer of Somebodies</u>.

Bruce has other short stories where we suspect the characters are on the spectrum, but we don't know for sure. "Disconnect" and "Chasing Rainbows," which were also published in <u>A Summer of Somebodies</u>, are two examples of these.

Given that Bruce wrote extensively about autism and the issues facing autistics in her novel <u>Glass On A Stick</u>, why would she bother to write additional fictional material? How could there be anything left to say after 205,000 words written about the subjects in the novel?

My answers to those questions would be that the themes running through the autistic world are many, and these many themes vary in complexity. There are more than enough themes to keep a single author writing many pieces of work.

<u>Glass On A Stick</u> was ambitious in scale and scope, encompassing an examination of autistics and self-diagnosed autistics both individually and in pairings and groupings. "Flux in Time and the Batman Blacklist Boogie Band" and "The Incredible Realtor", narrow the focus considerably and take a look at single self- diagnosed or diagnosed autistic characters individually.

While it may seem to people who haven't read either the book or the stories that the stories are a kind of shortchange, they are actually valuable in their own right. If we increase the power with which we look at something under a microscope's lens, we see it more clearly, and we learn more about it.

Such is the case in the two short stories.

In "Flux in Time," the character is self-diagnosed.

As I have stated in other articles, not all self-diagnosed autistics are detestable. But the one in the story seems to be. This one lies about in bed, thinking boy-thoughts, though he is a man. He lives with his parents, holds no job to speak of, believes himself to be a musician, though he hasn't produced anything of substance, and counts his days until his comic books arrive. He has an adversarial relationship with his parents. His floor is covered with dirty clothes and crawling with bugs. He is unkempt. -No, worse, he outright stinks.- He is a social anarchist of the laziest kind.

He also considers being an "autistic awarist" and using public speaking as an autistic awarist to get money.

Why would Elyse Bruce write something like this? Why would she paint self-diagnosed autistics in such a terrible light?

Well, the thing to remember here is that she is *not* painting self-diagnosed autistics (plural) in a terrible light. She is not even painting a self diagnosed autistic (singular) in a terrible light. What she has done is drawn a fictional character, pure and simple, and if there is any resemblance to a self-diagnosed autistic in real life, it is purely coincidental.

Yet we must admit that the law of probability would lead us to believe that a character like the one Bruce writes about *does* exist for real, possibly in a limited degree of proliferation. And if this is the case, then, like any other segment of society, sooner or later we would expect that it would fall under the gaze of a writer.

"Flux in Time" does not appear to be written as literary junk food, however. Some stories are like bad Grade B movies in the theatres. With those pieces of fiction, we're meant to throw tomatoes at the characters we hate. In Bruce's story, however, if we come to the end of it thinking that the character is repugnant, one moral that might be drawn is: The parents should do something to get the character to "man up." Another would be: If I see someone acting that way in real life, I should be less inclined to be sympathetic toward their laziness, and more inclined to motivate them to make something of themselves.

Further to the point of morals comes one that spans all of written history: Mainstream fiction, at the time that it is written, often reflects issues affecting society. If Bruce's story reflects an issue in society, and we don't like what she has shown us, who or what deserves the criticism? Bruce? Or the pervasiveness of the issue she writes about?

In "The Incredible Realtor" the oldest boy in the story, Brandon, AKA "Geektroid" is diagnosed on the spectrum. In this story, autism is arguably incidental to the story in the sense that any kid can fall victim to online predators the way Brandon does. But Brandon is not autistic in this story without purpose. Playing toward one of the perceived traits of autism, that autistics can sometimes be very gullible, Bruce shows us exactly how an autistic especially can fall victim to a predator. Taken in tandem with Glass On A Stick, we now begin to understand how one of Glass On A Stick's autistic characters, Emma Lynn, might fall into the clutches of ill intentioned self-diagnosed autistics.

When Brandon's mother contacts a friend to investigate the realtor who is stalking her son, we see another facet of autism: That of a parent of an autistic. While Brandon's mother's queries can be construed as interference and nosiness to begin with, in reality, she shows readers who do *not* have special needs kids, the extra lengths a parent of an autistic sometimes needs to go to to protect her child. This is a theme Bruce has not addressed before in other stories or even in her novel, which is ostensibly about a grandmother running a scam to gain funds for her alleged grandson who is supposedly autistic. In Glass On A Stick, Sarah Mae endangers her alleged grandchild by running a scam, whereas in "Realtor" Brandon's mother is clearly doing what is best to keep her son out of harm's way.

Getting back to autistics and autism in literature on a more general level, the complexity with which the aforementioned stories address autistic issues is not often seen in literature which has autism as its theme.

Part of the blame for the lack of good literary material may fall upon the big and little screen. Most people have seen *Rainman*. Many have heard about *Mozart and the Whale*. We are aware of the autistic characters in *St. Elsewhere, Parenthood*, and *Touch*.

Forgive me from being so critical, but those autistics whom I have had the good fortune to meet in real life do not bear much resemblance to those I see on television and in the movies. Similarly, they do not resemble realistically portrayed fictional autistic characters very much either.

If people read either my literary work or Elyse Bruce's literary work, and find themselves feeling positively or negatively emotional over the autistic elements included therein, they might ask themselves why they are so overcome. Is it because she and I as authors have succeeded in our attempt to be as true to autistics and autism as we could be?

If the answer is yes, then readers might do well to look for a better cut of literature going forward. Cast aside anything that is self-promoting, or which is designed to tug at your heartstrings in a sloppily melodramatic way.

One final point…

In keeping with the concept of literary archetypes, my stories and Elyse Bruce's works, are arguably structured on the "descent into the underworld" archetypal platform. The idea behind this archetype is that the characters descend into a figurative or literal underworld where they face others or face themselves, and then emerge from this underworld not necessarily unscathed, but changed.

"Flux in Time" presents us with an enigma in that the main character does not emerge from his brown study changed. Yet the story is relevant to today's times because this is a familiar problem we see with autistics and self-diagnosed autistics alike. Autism, for people of this type, becomes both a bane and a benefit for them. These types of people attribute success or lack of it to their autism. They ascribe their intelligence or intellectual shortcomings to their autism too. The result for people such as these is a sort of justified lethargy and laziness.

As we know, the world turns, and while it is seldom admirable to go against the world, it may be just as dishonorable to merely exist on it. The less proactive we are in trying to better ourselves, the less likely we are to become better people.

Can we plausibly argue to the contrary?

About Blogs

The next portion of this book is going to be about autistic authors, autism, and what can sometimes be called the lowest form of writing: The blog.

To be succinct: I am writing about bad blog entries about autism that are written by autistic authors.

Before I begin to talk to you about this topic, I want you to take a look at the voice I am using to write with right now. Also the style, diction, verbiage, etc. If you'll notice, the tone here is mostly informal, the language simple, the vocabulary something that's representative of the eighth grade reading level.

This is because I am not imparting something to you in a factual manner, as in a lecture, but in a casual form, as in a private chat, except in this case, rather than you and I having a reciprocal conversation, I am doing all the talking and you are doing all the listening, until later on, when you can write me letters about what I have said.

If I were writing to you online, instead of at my desk, I would be using an electronic format and delivery system, which means that I would be typing words with my keyboard, and posting them to a pre-designed online venue of my creation and ownership. You would then read my words from a laptop, PC, or other electronic device, and comment on them if you chose.

That's pretty much what a blog is: Simple words, written online, posted online, read online, responded to online.

A blog can take many forms. If you are like most people, you may have read a lot of blogs online. Some are factual, and read like books you'd buy in stores. Others are meant to be entertaining. Still others have a semi-private feel to them, and when we look at them, we feel almost like we are reading someone's personal secret diary.

In addition to my personal blog, at www.thomasdtaylor.wordpress.com, I write for the Midnight In Chicago blog at www.midnightinchicago.wordpress.com.

In regards to the MIC blog, it is what it is.

However, some days it is one thing, and some days it's another.

I have written many different posts on my communications with government officials, or charitable organizations, for example. Those posts were meant to inform, or to educate, and perhaps that was why, for some people, they made for dry reading. I gather that others *liked* the compact and efficient manner in which I reported my "stories" however.

Other posts have been commentaries, or editorials.

Still others are what I like to call "in between" posts. They are informative, and educational, but with an editorial flare. The material that you are reading now has its origins in a blog post, and I found as I composed the original material that it was impossible for me to use any other format for this particular topic.

And I am telling you all of this for what purpose?

Well, to show you that I understand that a blog is *just* a blog, and nothing more than a blog.

Did that point actually need to be stated?

Yes it did.

Why?

Because some people tend to make a bigger deal out of themselves *and* their blogs than they should. That's why.

I will elucidate further...

As I have mentioned in other posts, among my many different professional pursuits is writing. I have "published" in many forms, and the distribution of these various forms of publishing is equally varied. I have offered you that information because I believe it is important for an author/journalist/blogger to be true to one's readers. That means that one always show's oneself as one is and never pretends to be that which one isn't.

The addition of my book titles at the end of this publication, and my "resume" earlier on, is to demonstrate that I have some knowledge about writing generally, and so I feel qualified to give you my opinions about the topic of writing. It's also there for your benefit in a different sense: Is this just *anyone* who's offering an opinion? "No," you are to think. It is someone who has had some publishing experience.

If I am writing to you on a blog about other topics, I will not include my book titles because their inclusion is unnecessary and irrelevant. If I am blogging to you about some correspondence I've had with UNICEF, for example, my professional writing resume hardly matters. But here, in this book, it does matter in my opinion, and when this material was published in part in the "Autistics In Literature" article series on the MIC blog, it mattered also.

The thing is, if I were less than ethical, I would trumpet my resume everywhere, and use it as a vehicle to gain credence with readers, especially when whatever arguments I am asserting don't stand on their own. Have you ever noticed that some really terrible products have been hawked in commercial ads by celebrities? Unethical authors/journalists/bloggers do the same. "Look at me!" They will say. "Pay attention to me, and not so much in the believability of what I am telling you."

There are only a select few people who can get away with tacking their resume after their names. Three common examples are doctors (M.D.s), doctors (Ph.D.s), and people we commonly known to be associated with a certain profession, title, diagnosis, or combination thereof. Examples: Country Musician Taylor Swift, President Barack Obama, Autistic Author Temple Grandin.

The media can be guilty for ascribing labels to people who cannot and should not be labeled, and to people who do not want to be labeled. Donna Williams is much more than an author, and she is much more than autistic. Williams is an artist, a lecturer, and friend to many. Communicate with her and she will tell you that she is a person who has autism, not the embodiment of autism itself. Yet to the media, she is oftentimes, and more often than not "Autistic Author Donna Williams."

It seems that in this generation more people than ever have taken to creating their own image and then spend a great deal of time trying to get people to buy into that image. I believe that even though this is a very common practice, it may still be an unethical thing to do, because if you are not who you say you are, and if you have not accomplished what you say you have, what you are doing by promoting an "image" of yourself is inciting people to buy into an illusion.

Even authors are guilty of this kind of thing. Many of us have agents and publicists whose jobs it is to make us look good. Stephen King, if I am not mistaken, has written in "On Writing" that there were periods in his life where he was writing his books and stories with facial tissue stuck up his nose to stop the blood from pattering down on his fingers. Too much cocaine had caused his nose to bleed, you see. But we never knew of that, his family's intervention, or his subsequent rehabilitation until King himself told us about it.

That King is a very good author cannot be disputed. He has won a number of awards, has gotten much critical acclaim, and his sales are a testament to how much people like his writing. But as much as his books and his publishers do the selling for him, I believe a secondary reason for his great sales was and continues to be the fact that King has a likable personality, which he often displays during author interviews. My experience has been that people looking to buy something will more often buy something from people they like than from people they don't like.

But, if drug addiction is "bad," what if King's drug addiction had come to light at the worst possible moment? And what if there were other "bad" character traits that came to light at the same time? How would those revelations have affected his sales? How would those revelations affect his overall reputation?

Now it is true that no one is without sin. And it is true that many people engage in worse behaviors than King. Is it reasonable to expect that writers and authors should confess their sins to their readership in the same way that they would list out their resume?

I think it depends on what is being written about.

In King's case, it hardly matters whether he reveals an erstwhile drug addiction to us or not. He's a writer of fiction, and though there may be very important morals to impart in his stories, he is not necessarily a moralist per se, nor is he posing as someone whom he isn't. He is not, for example, an author writing anti-drug propaganda book about the drug trade, so he cannot be accused of being a hypocrite for revealing to us that he uses drugs.

Likewise, he does not do things like try to claim that the media he uses to impart his ideas is something that it isn't. When writing fiction, he says that it is fiction. When writing nonfiction, he identifies his words as such. If King had an underhanded motive, he writes deftly enough so that he *could* pass off fiction as nonfiction or vice versa. And if he had an agenda, and needed to appear authoritative to those he was trying to manipulate, he could pass himself off as someone he is not.

Fortunately, King *is* ethical, and I follow his ethics.

I have already revealed my credentials to show you who I am. Now I am going to tell you that when I publish *one* way, I do not claim to be publishing *another* way.

For example:

1. I have published seven books of fiction, but I am not writing fiction here in *this* book.
2. I may have edited someone else's books and supplied a few words for those books here and there, but I am *not* the author of *those* books.
3. I may have written editorial commentaries on various blogs, but those blogs were *not* newspapers, and I am *not* an editorial columnist.

Autistic bloggers are not exempt from deception. They will spend a great deal of time trying to create an image for themselves, and even more time trying to get people to buy into that image. And one way that makes them succeed in this deception, is when they pass off one type of media as another.

There are two online blog sites which ostensibly seem to be online newspapers. These are Huffington Post and Examiner.com. As I believe I have shown above, there are many different forms of publishing, and all forms are valid. While I have personal feelings about which forms of publishing are better than others, it is not my purpose specifically to lambaste the forms I consider less than stellar. My purpose is to point out that a particular form of publishing cannot be greater than what it is no matter how hard it tries.

Huffington Post and Examiner.com encourage people to write about particular topics in a journalistic fashion (as far as I can tell) but nowhere do they say —nor should they say- that their writers are professional journalists. To the extent that some of the writers write like professional journalists, and sound like professional journalists, they are journalists of a kind, but most of them are only amateur journalists because they are not writing for legitimate newspapers or magazines, and/or they do not have degrees in journalism.

To be a true journalist requires years in the making.

Someone who writes for The Washington Post is like a cup of coffee where the beans are hand picked, slow roasted, ground, and brewed. Someone who writes for Huffington Post is more like instant coffee. Still coffee, still consumable, but not as good.

This is not to slam any blogger or journalist, or write poorly about them. Nor is this a slam against Huffington Post or Examiner.com. They are what they are, and they do provide a useful service to their readership. I've read blog articles on both sites, and have learned much about many of the subjects being written about there.

But my opinion about those two publications and those who publish on them is –to my way of thinking- a valid opinion.

Another opinion I have is that it seems like people in the autism world who write on those sites call themselves journalists, or, even worse "autistic journalists."

Now granted, if Huffington Post and Examiner.com are journals, then the people who write for them are journalists. But if you ask me what a journalist actually is –and if you ask almost anyone else- the answer would be that a journalist is someone who writes for a publication that is indisputably a journal. Publications like The Washington Post, The New York Times, The Wall Street Journal, Time Magazine, Newsweek, and even Good Housekeeping and Rolling Stone Magazine are all journals.

Those publications have a history. They are commonly seen as respected publications, and those people who publish in them are commonly seen as journalists.

Now, it is theoretically possible for a blog to call itself a journal, I suppose. But if I am publishing in a blog as a journalist, ought I not to have the same qualifications as a journalist who writes for a recognized *traditional* journal? And if a blog that purports to be a journal does not have qualified journalists writing for it, can we say that such a blog upholds itself to a similar standard of integrity that other journals have? We can't say that, because other journals have staff with higher qualifications.

But if these arguments don't sway you, the legal system's view of blogs surely will. At the time of this writing, in most countries, if not in all countries, courts do not recognize blogs as journals, nor do they respect the right of blogs to protect the names of anonymous sources.

All these words that I have written up until now have been written for the purpose of making a single point: Though journalists can be bloggers, not all bloggers can be journalists. Ergo, when a blogger presents themselves as a journalist, try to find out what their qualifications as a journalist actually are, and don't be so quick to call them a journalist if all they are doing is writing for something like Examiner.com or Huffington Post.

To call oneself a journalist when one has no established qualifications is "bad", but to tack the "autistic" qualifier onto title is worse in my opinion, and potentially more misleading.

Assuming the "autistic journalist" actually has autism and is not self-diagnosed, why should the fact that someone has autism make them *qualified* to write about autism and bill themselves as an autistic journalist?

On the surface, it makes perfect sense. A person has autism. They know what it is to live with autism. They are therefore qualified to write about autism.

But what if the journalist didn't have autism? What if the journalist had alcoholism? How would it sound to your ears if you read

"The following article is from alcoholic journalist John Doe."

Or

"Journalist Richard Roe has been an alcoholic all his life…"

Or

"Today's news comes from Jane Doe, who provides a view of the world through a drunkard's eye."

Would we take any of those authors seriously? Perhaps, if they were talking about alcoholism we would, but it still sounds…well…kind of silly.

Why then, do we take "autistic journalists" seriously?

I will grudgingly admit that sometimes when people with autism write about autism, their diagnosis gives them some degree of authority on the subject, but as I have said before regarding autistic authors in general, my firm belief is that just having autism does not necessarily qualify someone to write about the topic.

In the first place, most people who write blogs are just that: Bloggers. This holds true whether they have a diagnosis or not. And because they are blogging, rather than writing as journalists, what they write should be taken in by us the same way we would consume fast food: It's pleasing, it tastes good, but it's not necessarily what's best for us.

In the second place, one's qualifications need to be taken into consideration as well.

I have stated *ad nauseum* that I have listed out a bunch of things I've done which I feel qualify me to talk about publishing. I have *not* listed out my diplomas, degrees, and awards. Hardly necessary, in my opinion. I never said I was a journalist. All I said was that I was an author, and I can say that because I have written and published seven books, some short stories, and some other things of note.

But if I wanted to say I was a journalist, I would first have to produce some evidence that I write or wrote for an actual journal, and, barring that, prove that I have a degree in journalism from an accredited college or university.

Here I will get into legal trouble if I start listing out the names of colleges and universities specifically, but let me just say that an accredited school is one that can be said to be recognized by certain organizations as being legitimate, and that has academic programs that meet certain standards. These programs have classes that are taught by qualified educators with proven credentials.

In the past decade or so, new "colleges" and "universities" have sprung up which look like accredited colleges and universities, and have programs like accredited colleges and universities, but do not meet the standards that are met by accredited colleges and universities. Try to transfer your credits from one of these places to an accredited college or university and you will not succeed.

In recent years, the line has been blurred between accredited and unaccredited schools even further, because the unaccredited schools have colluded together to form their own accreditation programs and organizations. Thus these new colleges and universities can *claim* to be accredited, but still can be substandard in comparison with historically proven accredited colleges and universities.

So, if a person says they have a degree in journalism from XXXX college or university, the degree they are waving in your face might not be worth the paper it's written on. That is something you have to investigate as a reader.

But even if you have done the homework, and discovered that the person whose writing you're reading is autistic, and has a journalism degree from an accredited university, can you trust that what this person is writing is completely truthful?

The answer to that question in these cases is almost *always* no for two reasons:

1. Nothing that anyone writes is written without some kind of slant, no matter how unbiased they say they are or believe themselves to be, and
2. Sometimes people have a specific agenda.

I have been watching autistic advocates online for a very long time now, and what I notice is that some of the larger (and most notorious) autism organizations infiltrate the online media and get published by it the way a bunch of amateur chefs will befoul a ceiling with pasta. They know that if there are a lot of people throwing a lot of sticky stuff, there's a good chance that no matter how much might fall off the ceiling, *something* thrown by *someone* will stick.

Autism self advocacy organizations in particular might have *dozens* of their members writing for Examiner.com and Huffington Post. Some will purposely assail the opinions of their fellow members in a realistic looking but contrived argument meant to lead the readership to a consensus and a conclusion. Other times, these same people and their organization's fellow members/bloggers may write similar sounding pieces on a particular topic to make it appear that a majority of the "journalistic" opinion supports a certain viewpoint.

It's all a coordinated effort, and it's all done to mislead.

The are many reasons autism self advocacy organizations might have to mislead people:

1. They want to increase their rankings in search engines by having their organization mentioned as many times as possible on the web.
2. They want to promote their organizations to attract a larger membership.
3. They want to get people to sign a petition *en masse*.
4. They have a political agenda, such as trying to get legislation passed, and want to swamp the net with their agenda.
5. They want to incite the autism community at large to act on an issue in a manner that is ultimately favorable to them.
6. They want to attack a sector of the autism community and make it look like they hold the majority of the public support.
7. They want to make people believe that the members of their organization are noted and/or prominent journalists to raise the standing of the organization in the eyes of the media, potential new members and also its enemies.
8. They want to make legislators believe that because of their supposed breadth of impact on the population at large, they are a viable political entity with significant influence.
9. By encouraging comments to their articles, they can gather intelligence about their supporters and dissenters, such as email addresses and IP addresses. (They can use this information later to either recruit people or bully them.)
10. By touting themselves as "authorities" in the areas they are talking about, there is an implied threat that if you disagree with them, there may be repercussions.

It's interesting to note that if you continually review the "board" profiles of some of the board of directors for many of these self-advocacy organizations, you will find that someone's profile might start out saying "Jane Doe is a self-diagnosed fast food restaurant employee who aspires to be an autistic author…"and over the course of months or years, this profile winds up changing little by little until it reads "Jane Doe is an autistic journalist who writes for <u>Huffington Post</u>.…"

In the intervening time, if you listen to Jane Doe rant and rave in a chat room, or if you communicate with her via email, you will discover that not only has she been fired from that fast food restaurant job, but she has been fired from many other jobs as well, and all of her attempts to get diagnosed autistic have resulted in her being diagnosed with bipolar disorder. But all that isn't mentioned in the final biographical send up. When you go on the autistic self advocacy organization's website, what you will read is "Jane Doe is an autistic journalist who writes for <u>Huffington Post</u>..."

I know someone who once wrote to each advisory board member of an organization individually, challenging the activities of some of its staff. The result was a denial and a shirking of responsibility by each advisory board member. The advisory board claimed they were not responsible for the activities of their staff outside the mandates of the organization. Regarding the resumes of the organization's staff, they claimed that they were not responsible for verifying the biographical or vocational information included therein, even when this information was posted on their website.

After this, the organization's staff stepped up their activities against the inquirer.

"Jane Doe is an autistic journalist..." sounds good to everyone who reads the biographical note, and for those people who wouldn't think to write for <u>Examiner.com</u> or <u>Huffington Post</u>, it sounds *really* good. The problem is, almost *anyone* can write for those two publications. If you don't believe me, fill out an application and give it a try. It's easy.

But it certainly sounds good for self-advocacy organizations to say they have a "journalist" on their board. And it certainly sounds good to someone reading the "journal" in question to read that the journalist whose work they're reading is a board member for an autistic self-advocacy organization.

People and organizations that engage in this behavior might see it as symbiosis. A person promotes himself a certain way, and an organization promotes the person the *same* way to the benefit of both the person and the organization.

But in a sense, it's mutual parasitism, with the person and the organization feeding off of one another so that each can be seen as being greater than what they are.

And as awestruck gullible readers, our organizational support and our donor dollars are the secondary food for these bugs.

Now then, what can we do to avoid being suckered?

Well, for one thing, that depends on how persistent or lazy you are in investigating the credentials of the person you believe to be a journalist. For another, if we are talking purely about journalism in the *autism* world, you ought to put yourself in the know about autistic politics.

The person who writes the article you're reading, whether it appears on a "journal" or a blog, could be any one of the following:

- ☐ Diagnosed
- ☐ Misdiagnosed
- ☐ Self-diagnosed
- ☐ In the process of getting a diagnosis
- ☐ Seeking a diagnosis
- ☐ A wannabee
- ☐ A parent of an autistic
- ☐ A sibling of an autistic
- ☐ A relative of an autistic
- ☐ A friend of an autistic
- ☐ A teacher
- ☐ A medical practitioner
- ☐ A researcher
- ☐ A reporter
- ☐ A curiosity seeker
- ☐ Neurotypical
- ☐ A Quack
- ☐ Someone who is trying to sell you something

If the person is autistic, they should be diagnosed with only *one* of the following, but may claim to be diagnosed with more than one of the following:

- Autism
- Asperger Syndrome
- Childhood Disintegrative Disorder
- Rhett Syndrome
- Pervasive Developmental Disorder Not Otherwise Specified?

(It should be noted that once the DSM V is commonly recognized, Autism Spectrum Disorder will be the *only* diagnosis an autistic person can have.)

Further questions to ask regarding the "autistic" author of the "article" you are reading:

- Is the "autistic" author high-functioning or low-functioning?
- Is the "autistic" author capable of functioning adequately in society, incapable of functioning adequately in society, or educably mentally handicapped?
- If the "autistic" author is low-functioning or educably mentally handicapped, is the article you are reading ghost written, and if so, by whom?
- Does the ghost written article properly reflect the intent of the "autistic" author?
- Does the "autistic" author have co-morbid diagnoses?
- Does the "autistic" author have allergies?
- Does the "autistic" author have synesthesia?
- Does the "autistic" author want to be treated or not?
- Does the "autistic" author want to be cured or not?

Regarding the author of the article (whether they are "autistic" or not):

- Does the author believe that autism is caused by vaccines?
- Does the author believe that autism is caused by mercury poisoning?
- Does the author believe that autism is caused by "Big Pharma" "vaccinating" or injecting people with autism? (Please note that some people will use the term "vaccinate" and "inject" interchangeably in this context.)
- Does the author believe that autism is caused by government "vaccinating" or injecting people with autism? (Please note that some people will use the term "vaccinate" and "inject" interchangeably in this context.)
- Does the author believe that autism is caused by genetics?
- Does the author believe that autism is the result of recessive Neanderthal genes becoming active?
- Does the author believe that autistics manifest genes that will eventually become active for everyone when the next phase of human evolution is complete?
- Does the author believe that autistics are alien-human hybrids?

Regarding the following issues:

- Is the author for or against ABA therapy?
- Is the author for or against chelation therapy?
- Is the author for or against gluten free therapy?
- Is the author for or against "Floortime"?
- Is the author for or against electroshock therapy?
- Is the author for or against restraints?
- Is the author for or against institutionalization?
- Is the author for or against an autism registry?
- Is the author for or against the sterilization of autistics?
- Is the author for or against a genetic test for autism?

- ☐ Is the author for or against weeding autistics out of the human genome through selective abortion?
- ☐ Is the author for or against abortion?
- ☐ Is the author for or against selective abortion?
- ☐ Is the author for or against the neurodiversity movement?
- ☐ Is the author for or against pushing the United Nations to grant autistics minority status?
- ☐ Is the author for or against the consolidation of the five DSM IV autistic spectrum disorders into one designation in the DSM V?

More important questions:

- ☐ Does the author like neurotypicals, hate neurotypicals, or hate neurotypicals but support the neurodiversity movement?
- ☐ Does the author support the idea that autism is a diagnosis?
- ☐ Does the author support the idea that autism is a difference, not a diagnosis?
- ☐ Does the author support the idea that autism is a disease, and not a difference or a diagnosis?
- ☐ Does the author support the idea that autism is a mental disorder?
- ☐ Does the author support the idea that autism is none of the above, but that autistics are really a minority group?
- ☐ Does the author support the idea that autistics are a separate race?

Some *very* important questions:

- ☐ Is the author morally conservative or liberal?
- ☐ What is the author's religion?
- ☐ What is the author's religious denomination?
- ☐ What are the author's political leanings?
- ☐ What autistic movements has the author supported or not supported?

- What petitions has the author signed, not signed, or refused to sign?
- What autistic alliances are the author affiliated with?
- What autistic organizations does the author belong to?
- If the author belongs to an autistic organization, what is their position within that organization?
- What government organizations is the author affiliated with?
- Who are the author's friends in the online and offline autism world?
- Has the author been arrested for illegal activity that could be linked to their autistic political views?

These questions are a fraction of what you should ask yourself before you elect to read something that is written by an "autistic journalist" (and an autistic blogger, podcaster, editorialist, autobiographer, or author, for that matter). And if you have forgotten why you should be asking these questions about autistic journalists and bloggers specifically, let's review a little....

1. Journalists can be bloggers, but not all bloggers are journalists.
2. Blogs can be journals, but most blogs aren't journals.
3. Many who call themselves journalists do not write for true journals and do not have journalistic credentials.
4. Some who call themselves "autistic journalists" are using the "autistic" descriptor to mislead people into believing they are more qualified to speak on the subject of autism that they are.
5. Both the academic qualifications and the organizational affiliations an "autistic journalist" may present to you may be suspect.
6. Many "autistic journalists" have agendas and ulterior motives for writing what they write.

And all of these six points, plus the questions I've asked, lead me to ask you: With so much doubt revolving around "autistic journalists", why would you want to risk reading what they have to say about autism? If you want material that is more trustworthy, your best bet is to read the actual research that has been done regarding autism. Or read the material published by recognized and respected autistics who have already established their credentials and demonstrated their integrity.

Mostly, trust your gut.

If something doesn't feel right, it probably isn't.

I am now going to ask perhaps the *most* important question of all, and it should be asked of anyone who purports to be on the spectrum, and who writes material that is intended to be read by someone else, whether this material is an editorial, a magazine article, a book, or a blog.

- ☐ Is there any evidence to suggest that he author whose work you are reading is part of an autistic supremacist group?

This last question may seem paranoid and unwarranted. However, if you have read this far, you may be thinking that some of the beliefs and behaviors displayed by some autistics seem very similar to those often displayed by supremacist groups.

Unfortunately, your intuition has not failed you. There are indeed people and groups who do believe that autistics are superior to all of mankind, and that it is the destiny of those with autism to rule the world. It sounds completely ridiculous on the surface, but when one considers that there are many famous people with autism, and that rumors of Thomas Edison, Henry Ford, and Albert Einstein's supposed autism abound, one can see how some autistics would believe themselves to come from superior genetic stock.

There are forums rife with hate speech against neurotypicals, and talk of how society should be structured and regimented a certain way, with autistics in control "for the betterment of mankind." Given that some of the people spouting this garbage hold college degrees, their language may sound compelling if not convincing, and the manner in which they draw you around to their way of thinking may be quite scholarly. Yet do not be fooled. These pronouncements sound startlingly similar to Adolf Hitler's Nazi propaganda.

The intrigue becomes more entangled when a member of one "faction" claims to be a member of another "faction" to torpedo an agenda. Many pro-vaxers, for example, will claim to be anti-vaxers, and deliberately troll online forums as anti-vaxers to get all anti-vaxers thrown off of those forums. Taking this one step further, a pro-vaxer might, as a "journalist" take the side of an anti-vaxer and deliberately write inflammatory stories, or stories with spurious content in an effort to make anti-vaxers look mentally unstable and uneducated.

The fact is, without having circulated in many different sectors of the online and offline autism community for an extended period of time, a person would be hard-pressed to know who is, or who is not a reliable and trustworthy author, and whether or not an author's motives are earnest and legitimate.

Here I am presented with a dilemma. Should I or shouldn't I list out the people and organizations which I believe to be suspect. The answer to that question must be no. Readers need to determine for themselves which people and organizations they deem "good" or "bad." For me to cite people and organizations specifically would provide an editorial slant which might influence people positively or negatively, but which might have negative repercussions for them either way.

Nonfiction

Autistic nonfiction can be just as guilty as autistic blogging in trying to push an agenda on its readers. Further, nonfiction can actually come across as more credible than any other mode of writing for the simple reason that emotional arguments are usually absent, and "support documentation" can be substituted to back up one's assertions.

Can the works cited be trusted in such circumstances? Yes and no. It depends on the works themselves, who wrote them, and how they are being used.

Often times credible and respected sources may be cited, but comments from those sources may be cherry-picked to support a different kind of argument than the source documents make.

Adding to the overall problem, with the proliferation of "autistic authors" comes a whole new list of new "sources" which may be quoted, and if any of these "autistic authors" have an agenda, or if they are poor researchers, they hardly qualify as sources.

What is one way an unethical autistic author can become a "source?"

Well, as with blogging, many "authors" from one organization with an agenda can now publish books on the same topic. If these authors publish their books in succession, each new author can quote the previous one, thereby giving credibility to an otherwise incredible "source."

This is how "authorities" on autism are "made" in many instances. But keeping in mind that these "authorities" may be no more knowledgeable about the subjects they are writing about than the readers who buy their books, it is important to research the authors themselves and find out more about them. The same questions that I suggested readers ask about bloggers and "journalists" should be asked about authors of nonfiction.

You will find many different agendas pushed through nonfiction, and you will find many specious sources to back up the theses of the authors. One of the more popular specious sources backs up the repeatedly disproved idea that vaccines cause autism.

Andrew Wakefield and his study are most often quoted as "sources," but many times absent from books that push this vaccines-cause-autism agenda are counterarguments, such as the fact that Wakefield was sanctioned, his medical license was revoked, and his research was disproved.

It would behoove readers of autistic nonfiction to be less trusting than they would be if they were reading books on some other kind of disorder or disability. There are of course many trustworthy authors of nonfiction that has autism as its main topic. Dr. Tony Attwood, M.S. Garnett, Simon Baron-Cohen, Michelle Dawson, Dr. Peter Szatmari, and Dr. Laurent Mottron

(M.D., Ph.D.) are just a few names that can be trusted, for example. But for each of those names, there may be dozens that cannot be trusted at all.

Just because someone publishes a book, appears at a convention, releases self-help audio tapes, is interviewed on podcasts, etc., doesn't mean they are a reputable author of nonfiction. Only the research they use to back up their argument matters. If the research is shoddy, or if it is used unethically, or if it used contrary to how it was intended, don't trust it as a "source."

The other thing readers should do is to educate themselves about autism research and autism researchers generally. I mentioned a name that is familiar to me, but perhaps not familiar to you: Dr. Laurent Mottron (M.D., Ph.D.). Who is he?

Among other things, he is:

1. Head Research Chair in Autism Cognitive Neuroscience at the University of Montreal
2. Scientific Director of the Centre for Excellence in Pervasive and Developmental Problems, University of Montreal
3. Tenured Professor, Department of Psychiatry, University of Montreal

What has he done?
Well.... Look it up!

Audio books and Podcasts

Audio books have been a popular form of publishing for some time. I like them, although to date, there has never been an audio book that I thought was better than the book itself.

One of my favorite audio books is Stephen King's "The Mist." Originally published as an enjoyable story in King's Skeleton Crew, the audio book adds sound effects, ostensibly to enhance the feel of the story. Whereas before we had to imagine everything, the audio book changed things in that:

1. We got to hear actors playing the part of our favorite characters
2. We got to hear background foley to get a better sense of setting
3. We got to hear the monstrous creatures

Standing on its own, the audio book is fine, but when juxtaposed with the printed story, the audio book was inferior in my opinion. My mind had already developed voices for the characters, and the audio book changed them. I had already imagined background noises, and the ones in the audio book were not quite like I heard in my mind. I had already imagined what the monsters sounded like, but the audio book gave me different sounds for them.

Perhaps it is because I am an author of horror myself, but when I read "The Mist" all by itself, my mind filled in all the blanks with more skill than what ever could have been injected into any audio book version of story, let alone the version I listened to.

The movie adaptation of "The Mist" can be complimented for its being fairly loyal to the original story, with minor variations and omissions doing little to take away from author intent. Disappointing, however, was the traumatic ending, which was present neither in the story nor the audio book. But what really made the movie thrilling and at the same time disappointing were qualities we can attribute to the medium itself:

1. We got to see the characters
2. We got to see the setting
3. We got to see the monstrous creatures

You see, having read the story, and having listened to the audio book multiple times, I was now faced with having to train my mind to be open-minded once more. Everyone and everything were once there for me in my mind in glaring detail. Now I had to erase my mental images of what the characters might look like, what the setting might look like, what the monsters might look like. And ultimately, after doing a comparison/contrast, I can tell you that while some of the movie jived with what my imagination had come up with, not all of it did.

While the movie does crystallize certain aspects of the book in our minds, it also nullifies much of what we may have previously imagined while reading the book. Likewise, while the audio book could be seen as a version of "The Mist" that falls halfway between the written story and the movie, it also detracts from the written story, because it dulls the imagination too.

Audio books and movies, it can be said, thwart our ability to interpret a written story in our own way, and they insert into our minds what the producer -not necessarily the author- wants us to take away from whatever form of the story that is presented to us.

You can see how I have illustrated how different forms of media can influence us in different ways.

But now imagine if we experienced *only* the audio book, or *only* the movie, and *not* the book? Would we be able to have an accurate sense of what the book was like given what the audio book "told" us, or what the movie "showed" us?

Audio books, which are a form of publishing in themselves, are a perfectly valid medium, I think, particularly when they are used for fiction. As much as I dislike the shortcomings of that particular form of media, they can still be quite entertaining. I have a different opinion, however, of audio books when they are being used for nonfiction. For me to explain why, I have to talk about H.G. Wells' War of the Worlds for a little while.

Many people have read H.G Wells's War of the Worlds, an interesting science fiction/fantasy novel that might have scared some readers when it was first issued, and might still scare people today. What followed from the original publication of the book was Orson Welles's excellent radio play (War of the Worlds) as well as a string of movie versions of varying quality. (I'm not even going to address the musical versions.)

My least favorite movie version is the one with Tom Cruise, though the special effects are good

In the book, the creatures from Mars land on Earth and construct their own instruments of destruction. In the movie version where Cruise plays the hero, the tripods are already buried beneath the surface of the Earth. When the aliens are shot to our planet via a sort of space lightning, they get into the machines and begin their annihilation of mankind.

But if the machines were buried hundreds if not thousands of years earlier, why did the aliens pick the modern era, when there were over seven billion people on Earth, to begin their conquest instead of when the population was much smaller, easier to find, and less able to defend themselves?

Further, if the aliens had been watching the Earth, waiting for the perfect moment to strike, did they not notice disease while they were doing their watching? Why didn't they ever send a probe to Earth to gather data about possible microscopic threats to them? Wasn't there anything like a monitoring device in their pre-positioned machines that might sense microorganisms which could prove lethal to the aliens? Didn't the aliens stop to think that bacteria might be their undoing in their battle for the Earth? Why didn't they develop an antibiotic to protect their troops, and administer that antibiotic to them before they were beamed to our planet?

Admittedly, we cannot blame the producer of the Tom Cruise version of War of the Worlds for the problem of the bacteria. Wells made the alien's lack of knowledge about bacteria the reason for their downfall. It only makes sense for the producer to carry that forward into the movie. Yet it's still unbelievable in the movie that an advanced civilization can bury tripods in the sand long before humans populate the Earth, and send their people from Mars to Earth via lightning strikes, but it couldn't figure out that there might be tiny organisms on the Earth that could destroy them.

The errors in this and other War of the Worlds movies we can excuse. As viewers, we understand that there will be omissions, interpretations, etc., that will cause a film to be different from a book. Producers, directors, and actors take liberties in films quite often. It's just the way it is.

One thing that is less excusable, however, was they manner in which Orson Welles's radioplay was done. Many listeners who tuned in during the middle of the broadcast, and who weren't familiar with <u>War of the Worlds</u>, actually believed the Earth was really being invaded by creatures from space.

Having heard the radioplay from beginning to end many times (I actually own a copy of it) I can see how, in that time in history, a person might have been snookered. The way Welles arranged things, supposed "regular programming" was interrupted by "bulletins" which gave "breaking news" and the "updates" on the supposed invasion of Earth by Martians. These "bulletins" and "updates" were given by authoritative sounding "reporters" to the listener in the same brisk and brusque manner of the period. "Reports" from supposed witnesses were broadcast also, and the background noises (which were really studio produced sound effects) lent an extra layer of "truth" to the whole thing. To add even *more* authenticity, a report would periodically get cut off, thereby forcing listeners to assume that on-the-spot "reporters" had been killed.

You can see here how it is that pure fiction broadcast over the radio can be made to seem like absolute reality if the formatting and staging are perfect. And as I have also demonstrated, you can see also how a movie could have huge plot flaws and still be a "blockbuster."

Today, podcasts have taken the place of radioplays. And movies still exist to "take liberties" with written books. With the right equipment and software any person could make up a podcast not dissimilar to the radioplay Welles made up decades ago, or they could make a movie to rival the Cruise version of <u>War of the Worlds</u>.

Think of the implications of that when it applies to nonfiction. Think of the implications of that when it applies to nonfiction that has autism as its main topic.

The public's gullibility has not lessened as quickly as technology has matured. People are not savvy enough to understand that something produced in someone's basement could sound and/or look very professional, but may really be a production that is meant to deceive. This is why I urge caution to anyone who normally trusts a podcast or a an audio book without first stopping to check who made the production, and without first stopping to investigate why the production was made.

As someone who has written and co-written many podcasts for Midnight In Chicago, I have taken great care to make them fact-based, with sources quoted and cited so listeners can review anything I say. The website where the podcasts are posted, www.podomatic.com, has terms of use that must be adhered to, but Elyse Bruce and I have put rules of our own into effect that go beyond those on www.podomatic.com. At www.autism.podomatic.com, you will find cheerful podcasters, but you will not find ones who will try to hypnotize you, or try to subtly or subliminally influence you. In other words, while we try to sound pleasant, we do not use tones in our voices or other gimmicks to try to get you to believe something that you would not so easy believe if you were just reading it.

Audio books can have an even more powerfully influential effect on you that podcasts do. If you are listening to an audio book that is nonfiction, chances are you will be listening to one voice -without background noise or foley- for the entire recording. Listen long enough and you may find yourself falling into a state of mind that is more suggestible than if you were having a give and take conversation with people.

If you don't believe me, try to think back to times in history when whole nations were rallied to a cause. Where people have been rallied most effectively, it was usually in a situation where they were enclosed in a building or stadium, and where one lone speaker spoke on and on for a very long period of time, slowly bringing everyone to a consensus. People would become more rapt with attention with each passing minute until finally, the final words were given, and whether those words were The Final Solution (Holocaust) or "Kamikaze! Kamikaze! Kamikaze!" or what have you, the people approved!

Books afford you the opportunity to go back and re-read what you have read. While you may be able to do the same with audio books and podcasts, you may not be so inclined, because

1. It is instinctual in us not to interrupt people while they are still talking
2. We are trained not to ask questions until people are finished speaking

3. It may simply be inconvenient to rewind or replay a
    portion of the recording

In audio books and podcasts, a person's voice, or the speed at which they speak, can distract us and keep us from thinking logically, but with a book, there is nothing but words on a page. If we do not understand a word in a recording, we may not have time to dig out a dictionary to find out what it means, but when we are reading a book, time affords us the opportunity to get out a dictionary and educate ourselves.

In time, I may elect to issue my fiction and nonfiction books in audio book format. If or when I do so, I will make sure the content therein will be true to the original text in the books. Can you trust authors will who write about autistics and autism will do the same?

There are many "autistic radio" shows out there that are really just podcasts, scripted podcasts, or audio books in podcast format. Some of these are produced by people who have ulterior motives. Again, I urge people to check the credentials of the people who write audio books and podcasts about autism, and I urge you to ask questions about their motives.

Winding Things Up

Going forward, I hope that everyone who reads this book will begin to cast a more critical eye on the plethora of autistic literary material out there. We are not educating ourselves about autism when we read material that is designed to deceive. We are not learning anything about autism if the source is questionable or disreputable. We are not learning anything about autism if the people teaching you about it have a vested interest in skewing the subject matter in their favor.

With all of that said, I would be remiss if I did not critique this very book. Literature, as we know, includes nonfiction, and that is what this book is.

When it is published, what will it be, exactly?

Can we call it a reference book?

Hardly. While it makes reference to people, periodicals, and publications, and while it tackles the subject of autistics and autism in literature, and autistic authors, it hardly encompasses every element of the topic, nor is the examination of the topic done in much depth.

In typical nonfiction, specific sources are usually cited, bibliographies are given, and the tone of the writing is generally more neutral. Equal dedication is usually provided to the discussion of topics included in the publication, but I have only touched upon certain topics, such as nonfiction.

No, what I have written here is largely an opinion piece or commentary, and I am not going to promote it as anything other than that. Similar to Stephen King's <u>Danse Macabre</u> and his <u>On Writing</u>, in its informality, it is also similar to those books in that it takes the view of an author talking about (in part) literature. In King's case, in his two books he is talking about horror as a genre, and writing, respectively. In my case, I am talking about autistics and autism in literature, both as a type of genre, and in terms of how autistics and non-autistics create literature and are portrayed in literature.

As I have indicated earlier on in this book, I believe the number of different ways I have been published qualifies me as an author, and the extent to which I have circulated in the online and offline autistic community qualifies me to write on the subjects of autistic authors, and autistics and autism in literature.

Being qualified means (to me at least) being honest, and so I must honestly say that this book is not meant to be a formal thesis or treatise (however formally or informally written), but merely an exploration. I should hope that other reputable and serious-minded authors take this publication and view it as a springboard to explore the topic further. To further that endeavor, his book will be offered at a reasonable price so that it might reach the widest possible audience.

At this time in history, 2013, it is important to recognize that the availability and convenience of the internet makes it possible for everyone who uses it to make available for reading their own views about autism. I have made some observations about what I have seen. As time goes on, what we *all* have seen will recede into the background as new material is published. I should think the nature of the published materials will naturally evolve, either in a forward or backward direction, or both.

Thus we cannot draw any conclusions, or even generalizations, about autistic authors and autistics and autism in literature at present, except to say that by gradations, it has grown and continues to grow out of primitivism.

Afterword

As I finish, I would like to state that I have not cited much material from these "good" authors should not in any way imply that they or what they have written is "bad." Their omission was due primarily to my desire to keep this book as compact as possible, and also due to the accessibility of the authors and/or their writing.

Having not required Stephen King's opinions about his autistic character in The Regulators and his mentally disabled character in Dreamcatcher, but only a general synopsis and some general supplementary material, I cited those works, although without using specific quotations. My own writing was of course easily accessible to me as were my thoughts and motives behind the writing. Elyse Bruce has graciously allowed me to address her novel Glass On A Stick, and her "Flux in Time and the Batman Blacklist Boogie Band," and "The Incredible Realtor" stories, and has provided me with valuable input about their drafting.

While it is regrettable that there has been so much negativity associated with "autistic" authors and the material that has been published that has "autistic" characters or "autism" as its core components, I foresee a time when the better authors and the better material will begin to have the prominence and staying power as do authors and literature in regular and accepted literary genres. When that happens, it may be worthwhile to pick up the threads of this commentary and continue.

In time, I may also write other books that pertain to autism generally.

Until then, thanks for reading.

Partial Annotated List of Works Cited

The following people, organizations, works or sources were cited, referenced, or discussed in passing or at length in this publication and have been included here because the author feels they may be of some interest to the reader. This list does not encompass all citations in this publication. Inclusion or omission of people, organizations, works, or sources does not constitute any endorsement or lack thereof. Supplementary information has been included where the author though it might be helpful or useful to the reader.

People:

Dr. Tony Attwood
Simon Baron Cohen
Bozo the Clown
Tom Cruise
Elyse Bruce
Jesus Christ
Edan Dagan
Claire Danes
Michelle Dawson
Thomas Edison
Albert Einstein
Henry Ford
M.S. Garnett
God
Temple Grandin
Adolf Hitler
Dustin Hoffman
Rock Hudson

Stephen King
Dr. Laurent Mottron, M.D., Ph.D.
President Barack Obama
Kim Peek
Taylor Swift
Dr. Peter Szatmari
Thomas D. Taylor
Andrew Wakefield
Orson Welles
H.G. Wells
Donna Williams

Organizations:

Autism Speaks
Big Pharma
Convention on the Rights of People with Disabilities
Government
Olympics
Midnight In Chicago (www.midnightinchicago.com)
Nazis
UNICEF
University of Montreal

Blogs:

Examiner.com
Huffington Post
The Midnight In Chicago blog
(www.midnightinchicago.wordpress.com)
The Thomas D. Taylor blog (www.thomasdtaylor.wordpress.com)

Periodicals

Good Housekeeping
The New York Times
Newsweek
Readers Digest
Rolling Stone Magazine

Time Magazine
The Wall Street Journal
The Washington Post

Publications:

By Elyse Bruce:

A Summer of Somebodies (Copyright 2012, Elyse Bruce)

"Chasing Rainbows" (Copyright 2012, Elyse Bruce. Published in A Summer of Somebodies)

"Disconnect" (Copyright 2012, Elyse Bruce. Published in A Summer of Somebodies)

"Flux in Time and the Batman Blacklist Boogie Band" (Copyright 2012, Elyse Bruce. Published in A Summer of Somebodies)

Glass on A Stick (Copyright 2012, Elyse Bruce)

"The Incredible Realtor" (Copyright 2012, Elyse Bruce. Published in A Summer of Somebodies)

By Edan Dagan:

The Aspergian Mythos

By Temple Grandin:

Emergence (Autobiography)

By Stephen King:

Bag of Bones (Novel)
Danse Macabre (Nonfiction)
Dreamcatcher (Novel)
IT (Novel)

"The Mist" (story)
The Mist (Audio book)
On Writing (Nonfiction)
The Regulators (Novel)
Salem's Lot (Novel)
Skeleton Crew (Short story anthology)
The Stand (Novel)

By Thomas D. Taylor:

Evil Creeps In: A Tale of Exorcism (Copyright 2011, 2012, Thomas D. Taylor)

Geo-13: The Lost Expedition (Copyright 2011, 2012, Thomas D. Taylor)

Geo-213: The Lost Stories (Copyright 2012, by Thomas D. Taylor

Ghostly Quintet: Five Tales of Ghosts, Apparitions, and the Beyond (Copyright 2013, Thomas D. Taylor)

"Little Green Men" (Copyright 2013, Thomas D. Taylor. Published in Ghostly Quintet: Five Tales of Ghosts, Apparitions, and the Beyond)

"The White Nurse" (Copyright 2013, Thomas D. Taylor. Published in Ghostly Quintet: Five Tales of Ghosts, Apparitions, and the Beyond)

By H.G. Wells:

War of the Worlds

Other:

Bible

DSM IV

(Diagnostic and Statistical Manual of Mental Disorders, 4th edition)

DSM V
(Diagnostic and Statistical Manual of Mental Disorders, 5th edition)

ICD 10
(International Statistical Classification of Diseases and Related Health Problems, 10th edition)

Movies:

The Mist
Mozart and the Whale
Rainman
Temple Grandin
War of the Worlds (with Tom Cruise)
Winchester 73

Musicals:

War of the Worlds

Radioplays:

War of the Worlds

Television:

Bozo's Circus
Parenthood
St. Elsewhere
Touch

Websites:

www.amazon.com
Aspergia (www.aspergia.com)

www.createspace.com
Midnight In Chicago www.midnightinchicago.com
www.podomatic.com
Midnight In Chicago Podcasts www.autism.podomatic.com
Wikipedia
YouTube

Other:

Aspie Quiz
Australian Scale for Asperger Syndrome

About the Author

Thomas D. Taylor is an author, an artist, a photographer, a songwriter, and (along with Elyse Bruce) Co-Creator of <u>Midnight In Chicago,</u> a 100% volunteer-run international initiative which raises funds and awareness for people with disabilities.

His short story "The Interview" won the First Place Fiction award in the 1991 edition of <u>Towers</u> literary magazine. Another of his stories, "A Grasshopper Cerebrates Humanity," was published in the same issue. In 2013, his political commentary, "Idle No More: A White Man Speaks," was published in <u>The First Perspective</u> magazine.

Taylor's artwork has sold worldwide. Taylor painted the front and back cover art for two of singer/songwriter Elyse Bruce's albums: <u>Midnight in Chicago,</u> and <u>Countdown to Midnight</u>. His photograph, "Library" appears on the cover of this publication.

Taylor is also responsible for co-writing three songs with Elyse Bruce: "Late Night In The Borough", "Somewhere In Detroit," and "How Do I Begin To Believe (Lying In The Arms Of My Judas)."

Other Books By Thomas D. Taylor

Science Fiction

Geo-213: The Lost Stories
Geo-213: The Lost Expedition

Horror

Evil Creeps In: A Tale of Exorcism
Deadly Duo: Two Stories of Death and Murder
Gruesome Triad: Three Stories of the Macabre
Grim Quatrain: Four Tales of Terror
Ghostly Quintet: Five Tales of Ghosts, Apparitions, and the
Beyond

www.ingramcontent.com/pod-product-compliance
Lightning Source LLC
Chambersburg PA
CBHW070536290526
45790CB00002B/515